Natural Herbal Remedies for Dogs

A Holistic Science-Backed Guide to Canine Herbalism—Safe DIY Remedies, Common Condition Protocols, and Vet-Friendly Tips to Keep Your Dog Thriving for Years to Come

Angela Lain

Copyright © 2025 by Angela Lain

All rights reserved.

No portion of this book may be reproduced in any form without written permission from the publisher or author, except as permitted by U.S. copyright law.

Contents

1. Introduction — 1
2. Foundations of Safe Canine Herbalism — 4
3. Getting Started—Your Herbal Toolkit and Sourcing Essentials — 28
4. Herbal Preparation Methods—DIY Remedies Made Simple — 44
5. Safe Dosage and Administration—Personalized for Every Pup — 59
6. Everyday Remedies for Common Canine Ailments — 71
7. Advanced Herbal Support for Chronic and "Left Out" Conditions — 87
8. Integration with Modern Pet Lifestyles — 106
9. Visual Reference Guides—Empowering Safe, Confident Decisions — 119
10. Real-Life Success Stories—Case Studies from Holistic Vets and Dog Parents — 137
11. Conclusion — 152

Introduction

It starts with that pit-in-your-stomach moment—the one where your dog, the furry heartbeat of your home, isn't feeling well. Maybe it's itchy skin that won't quit, digestion that's all over the place, or a sudden bout of anxiety that leaves both of you trembling. You've tried the vet, you've wandered the endless aisles of pet stores, and you've gone down countless rabbit holes on the internet, reading about "natural" remedies—only to find vague instructions, dosage confusion, or worse, warnings about toxicity. You just want to help your dog feel better. Safely. Naturally. Confidently. But the more you read, the more overwhelmed you become. Sound familiar?

You're not alone—and I'll let you in on something: that was me, too. Several years ago, I found myself sobbing on the kitchen floor with a handful of supplements and herbs, scared that I might hurt the dog I loved so dearly. I was doing my best, reading everything I could, but the fear of making a mistake with herbal remedies nearly paralyzed me. That fear turned into a mission. I refused to believe that compassionate, science-backed natural care for dogs had to be so confusing. I devoted years to learning from clinical herbalists, holistic vets, and peer-reviewed studies—and decided to turn everything I discovered into this one, clear, supportive guide.

If you've ever wondered: Can I really trust this advice? Is this plant safe for my dog's size? What's the right dose? What if something goes wrong? — you're in exactly the right place. This book grew out of hundreds of conversations with dog parents just like you. The pain points were always the same: uncertainty about safety, fear of doing harm, contradictory information from strangers on the internet, and the longing for a trusted resource that simply made sense. I see you—and this book was made for you.

Here's what you'll find inside: a comprehensive, beginner-friendly, science-based guide to herbal remedies specifically for dogs. No miracle claims. No mystery herbs you have to import. Just clear, confidence-building guidance rooted in research and enhanced by real-world experience. We'll unpack exactly how to choose, prepare, and deliver herbal remedies safely—complete with weight-specific dosage charts, visual guides, color-coded safety systems, and troubleshooting tools like flowcharts and red flag checklists, so you're never left guessing. You'll also read honest success stories from other dog parents who've gone down this very path—sometimes out of curiosity, sometimes as a last resort—and learned to care for their pups naturally and effectively.

You might be skeptical. That's healthy. You might be thinking, "Will this really work for my dog?" or, "I don't want to make a mistake." Those concerns are not only valid—they're welcomed here. Throughout the book, I'll show you how to navigate those doubts with evidence, step-by-step examples, input from licensed vets, and easy-to-follow visuals that support you every step of the way.

This book doesn't promise that herbs are the answer to everything. But it will show you how to use them as a powerful part of your dog's wellness toolkit—alongside good veterinary care. We'll focus only on safe, well-documented herbs, used correctly and responsibly, to address common canine concerns like anxiety, joint stiffness, digestive troubles, skin issues, immune support, and everyday maintenance. No advanced jargon. No lectures. No assumptions that you already know the difference between a tincture and a tea. Just friendly, empowering education that meets you exactly where you are.

By the time you finish, you'll know:

- How to confidently identify and select herbs based on your dog's specific issues

- How to make herbal remedies at home—or choose trusted premade options

- Exactly how much to give your dog based on weight and form (tea, tincture, powder, etc.)

- What signs to watch for (both positive effects and red flags)

- When herbs are appropriate—and when you need to head to the vet instead

- How to build a holistic, sustainable care plan that supports your dog over time

This isn't just a book. It's a companion on your journey—a non-judgmental guide in your corner that believes in your love for your dog, your willingness to learn, and your ability to get it right.

So take a breath. You've already taken the most important step: choosing to show up, curious and caring, for your dog's health. Let this book be your map. You're not alone anymore. And together, we're about to unlock the plant-powered potential within your reach—safely, clearly, and with heart.

Foundations of Safe Canine Herbalism

When embarking on a journey into the world of canine herbalism, safety must be our guiding principle. This chapter lays the foundation for navigating the rewarding—but sometimes complex—territory of integrating herbal remedies into your dog's wellness regimen. Before blending tinctures or steeping teas, we must understand the unique physiology of dogs, how herbs interact with their systems, and the critical factors that differentiate canine herbalism from human applications.

In this chapter, you'll discover the core principles that ensure herbs are used safely and effectively for dogs. We'll start by exploring the importance of species-specific considerations—recognizing that what's safe for humans or other animals may be harmful to a dog. You'll learn how to assess herb quality, understand dosage calculations tailored for canine bodies, and identify red flags for overuse or adverse reactions.

We'll also delve into basic canine anatomy and metabolism as it pertains to herbal use. With this foundational knowledge, you'll be equipped to make educated, confident decisions about incorporating herbs into your dog's care plan—working independently or in collaboration with a holistic or veterinary professional.

Whether you're a pet owner curious about natural approaches or an animal care provider seeking to add herbal tools to your skill set, this chapter sets the tone for responsible practice. Let's begin where all sound herbal work must—by placing safety, education, and respect for our canine companions at the heart of everything we do.

Decoding Dog-Safe vs. Toxic Herbs—A Visual Identification Guide

Navigating the world of herbs for canine wellness can feel like stepping into a botanical minefield. While many herbs offer incredible benefits for dogs—from calming nerves to aiding digestion—others can be dangerously toxic, even in trace amounts. Understanding which herbs are safe versus which should be strictly avoided is not only essential for your dog's health but also empowering for you as a responsible pet guardian.

It starts with recognizing the most commonly used herbs and distinguishing the helpful from the harmful. For example, chamomile, calendula, ginger, and parsley are widely used in natural dog remedies and are typically safe when used appropriately. To help identify these herbs, a visual reference chart with high-resolution photographs can be a game-changer. Each image includes key botanical details such as leaf shape, flower structure, and stem characteristics that allow for quick, at-a-glance recognition.

Dog-Safe Herbs

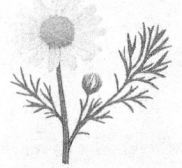

Chamomile
Feathery leaves, daisy-like flower

¼ tsp dried flower per 20 lbs (tea)

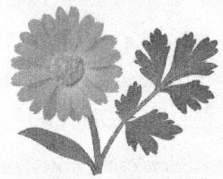

Calendula
Bright orange flower, lance-shaped leaves

Topical use or tea rinse

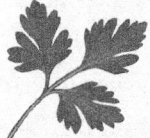

Parsley
Flat, lobed leaves ridged green stem

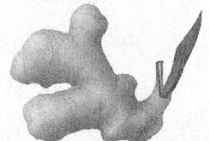

Ginger
Knobby rhizome, narrow, pointed leaf

Note Cristallalation is safe – reliquefy with gentle warming

In contrast, herbs like garlic, tea tree (Melaleuca alternifolia), and pennyroyal pose serious health risks to dogs—even in small doses. Garlic, though a staple in many human diets, can lead to anemia in dogs. Tea tree oil, popular in topical treatments, is highly toxic when ingested. Pennyroyal, often found in flea repellents, can cause liver failure. These dangerous herbs are featured in a corresponding toxicity chart, clearly differentiating them through visuals and quick facts that alert dog owners to proceed with caution.

Visual identification can be tricky, particularly when toxic and safe herbs look deceptively similar. That's why side-by-side photo comparisons are included to highlight such common confusions. For instance, the resemblance between safe mint (Mentha spp.) and toxic pennyroyal (Hedeoma pulegioides) can cause disastrous mix-ups. Leaf patterns, stem coloration, and even aroma cues are discussed to aid confident identification.

Toxic Herbs

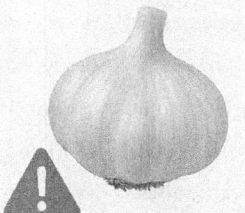

Garlic
Bulb
May cause vomiting,
weakness, collapse
Seek vet care

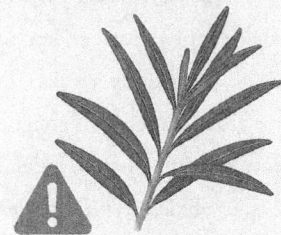

Tea Tree
(Melaleuca alternifolia)
Leaves
Drooling, weakness,
Immediate vet visit

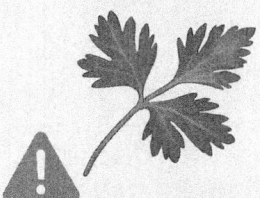

Pennyroyal
All parts
Can cause
vomiting, lethargy,
c failure

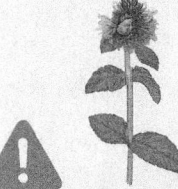

Pennyroyal
All parts
Can cause vomiting,
lethargy, liver failure
Contact vet at once

Additionally, you can tell the difference between fresh and dried herbs—a stumbling block for many. Dried herbs often lose their vibrant colors and unique textures, making them harder to identify. Tips for recognizing herbs from trusted herbal stores, farmers markets, or even your own garden are included, as well as guidance on labeling and storage to avoid accidental cross-contamination.

Mint vs. Pennyroyal

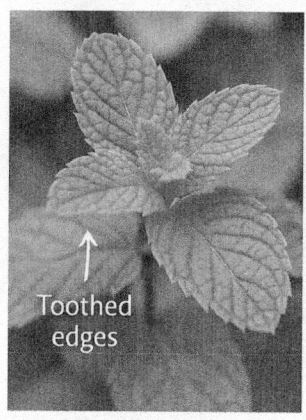

Toothed edges

Refreshing aroma

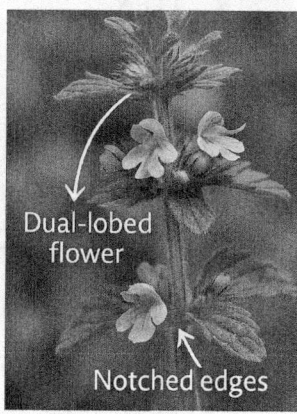

Dual-lobed flower

Notched edges

Liver shape

One of the most frequently cited concerns from pet parents is the overwhelming fear of poisoning their pets due to conflicting advice found online. It's not uncommon to find contradictory statements about a particular herb's safety, leading to anxiety and hesitation. To address this, look for clearly marked "Herb Lookalike Warnings" within your guide—visual callout boxes that spotlight particularly confusing herbs. These warnings offer specific cues that help dispel the doubt between friend and foe in your herb cache.

Fresh vs. Dried Herb Guide

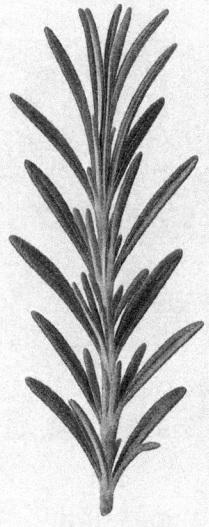
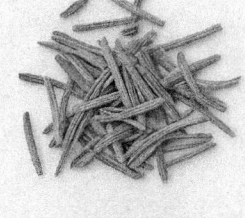
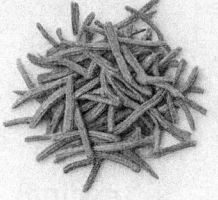

Fresh **Dried**

TIP: Look for shriveled leaves, muted color, lighter aroma

For urban and suburban readers, sourcing herbs safely can be a particular challenge. A "Safe Sourcing Checklist" is provided, offering criteria to evaluate vendors, determine growing methods (e.g., pesticide-free), and ensure proper labeling. This checklist makes it easy to vet local shops, online stores, and even community gardens, helping you source with confidence no matter where you live.

Safe Sourcing CHECKLIST

Evaluate Vendors

- Look for transparent sourcing info (farm name, location)
- Ask about 'harvesting methods and freshness
- Prefer small/local vendors who specialize in herbs

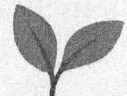

Growing Methods

- Choose pesticide-free or organic whenever possible
- Avoid herbs with artificial coloring or additives
- Check for certifications if USDA Organic, Non-GMO

Proper Labeling

- Labels should include:
  - Herb name
  - Common +/riet
  - Storage instructions
- Avoid unlabeled bulk bins unless from a trusted source

Where to Source

- Local Shops: Health food stores, herbal apothecaries
- Farmers Markets: Talk directly with growers
- Community Gardens: Verify ac ro pesticides

Empowering yourself with visual tools, botanical knowledge, and trusted references can eliminate guesswork and give you peace of mind. As you explore herbal wellness for your dog, remember that a little education goes a long way in protecting the furry members of your family. From confusion to confidence, this guide sets the foundation for safe, informed herbal care.

Science Meets Tradition—How Herbal Remedies Actually Work for Dogs

Herbal remedies for dogs may carry the weight of centuries-old tradition, but in modern times, their effectiveness is increasingly being understood through the lens of science. While these natural treatments were once dismissed as "old wives' tales," mounting research in veterinary science and pharmacognosy (the study of medicinal plants) is bridging the gap between ancestral wisdom and empirical evidence. To fully appreciate how herbal medicine works for canines, it's essential to explore both the physiological realities of dogs and the evolving scientific perspectives on plant-based therapies.

Dogs metabolize herbs differently than humans, owing to distinctions in digestive enzyme profiles, liver function, and organ sensitivities. For example, a dog's liver processes certain plant alkaloids more slowly than a human liver, which can amplify or prolong the herb's effect. Additionally, their shorter gastrointestinal tract can alter the absorption rate of some phytochemicals. When a dog consumes a herb like peppermint, its active compounds—such as menthol—are absorbed into the bloodstream and interact with organ systems like the gut and nervous system. In simplified terms, peppermint can relax smooth muscle tissue in a dog's intestines, easing minor digestive discomfort. Such interactions, while once entirely anecdotal, are now being modeled and measured in laboratory settings for greater precision and predictability.

Traditional herbal wisdom often aligns remarkably well with modern veterinary data. A compelling example is the use of chamomile for anxiety. Folk remedies have recommended chamomile tea for calming both humans and animals for generations. Scientifically, chamomile contains apigenin, a flavonoid compound that binds to the same receptors in the brain as some anti-anxiety drugs, promoting mild sedation. Veterinary studies further support its efficacy, though results vary based on dose and extract concentration. Another case is turmeric, frequently used in Ayurvedic medicine for inflammation. Recent peer-reviewed studies have highlighted curcumin—turmeric's active component—as a potential natural aid in managing joint pain and stiffness associated with canine arthritis, with some reporting reduced reliance on NSAIDs in dogs supplemented with curcumin under veterinary guidance.

Still, skepticism persists, and understandably so. Herbal remedies have often been promoted with enthusiastic anecdotal evidence without the rigorous standards of clinical research. However, this doesn't render them ineffective—it highlights the need for discernment. Not every plant suits every dog, and not all formulations are created equal. Holistic veterinarians, like Dr. Karen Becker, emphasize transparency and caution when using herbs: ""We see herbs as tools, not cures. Like pharmaceuticals, they need to be matched correctly to the patient, monitored, and adjusted as needed."" Clinical herbalists echo this, pointing out that documented efficacy and safety must guide herbal recommendations, particularly when used alongside conventional treatments.

Real-world examples often put a face to these statistics. Consider Luna, a ten-year-old Labrador retriever with recurring hot spots. After multiple rounds of antibiotics produced diminishing results, her caregiver tried calendula salve under holistic supervision. Calendula, traditionally used to soothe skin inflammation, has known antibacterial and wound-healing properties—confirmed in both laboratory and field studies. Within a week, Luna's sores showed significant improvement. However, not all dogs respond positively to botanical remedies. Factors like breed-specific metabolism, the dog's age, the severity of the condition, and even how the herbal remedy is prepared—whether as a tincture, tea, capsule, or topical application—can make the difference between success or frustration.

In the end, herbal medicine for dogs thrives at the intersection of science and tradition. It's a growing field that asks practitioners and pet parents alike to think holistically but act responsibly. By appreciating both the deep roots of herbal history and the modern studies that validate (or challenge) that wisdom, we can navigate this path with clarity, compassion, and confidence. As we move forward, understanding how to choose and administer herbs smartly will be the next logical step—one that ensures safety and maximizes benefit for our four-legged friends.

Understanding Contraindications and Red Flags in Canine Herbal Care

When using herbs to support your dog's health, it's essential to understand contraindications—specific situations where a remedy should not be used because it may cause harm. In plain terms, a contraindication is a reason to say "no" to a particular herb based on your dog's medical condition, age, breed, or other factors. Recognizing these red flags can be the difference between helping your dog and unintentionally causing discomfort or a dangerous reaction.

For example, licorice root—often praised for its anti-inflammatory and adrenal-supportive benefits in holistic medicine—poses a serious risk for dogs with heart disease or high blood pressure. This herb can cause sodium retention and increase blood pressure, which may worsen existing cardiovascular conditions. Similarly, herbs like black cohosh or pennyroyal, which may be safe for some adult dogs in very limited contexts, can be extremely toxic to pregnant dogs or nursing mothers.

Responding quickly to early warning signs of adverse reactions is another pillar of safe herbal use. While most dogs tolerate herbs well, knowing what mild, moderate, and severe reactions look like can empower you as a responsible pet guardian. Mild symptoms might include temporary digestive upset (like soft stools), increased itching, or a decrease in appetite shortly after starting a new herb. More moderate signs could include persistent vomiting, hives, swelling around the eyes or mouth, or lethargy. Severe red flags—requiring immediate veterinary care—include breathing difficulties, facial or throat swelling, seizures, bloody diarrhea, or collapse. Never ignore sudden changes in behavior or health following a new herbal introduction.

A handy way to stay proactive is to refer to visual symptom cues or maintain a reaction diary. Watching for reactions is particularly important during the first 72 hours after starting a new herbal regimen. Tracking subtle changes such as restlessness, panting, or skin changes often provides early signals that your dog's system may be rejecting the herb or metabolizing it poorly.

Choosing herbs safely also requires knowing which ones aren't suited for your dog's specific life stage or medical background. Puppies have developing livers that process substances differently, making them sensitive to even gentle herbs like valerian or echinacea. Senior dogs may have reduced organ function or be on prescribed medications that interact poorly with herbs such as ginkgo biloba or milk thistle. Pregnant and lactating dogs must be handled especially carefully—herbs like dong quai or goldenseal may stimulate uterine contractions or affect milk production. Brachycephalic breeds (like Bulldogs or Pugs) with respiratory sensitivities should avoid mucilaginous herbs that may thicken mucous secretions, such as marshmallow root.

To help you make informed choices, maintain a checklist that matches herbs to your dog's age, breed-specific concerns, and existing health conditions. Keep this list nearby when researching or shopping for herbal products. Prioritize professional consultation before adding new herbs—especially if your dog is already on any form of medication.

One core principle to always remember: "When in Doubt, Leave It Out." If a certain herb's safety for your dog isn't crystal clear or you're uncertain about dosage or interactions, it's better not to use it at all. Guesswork has no role in canine wellness. Instead, test herbs cautiously with a step-by-step approach: introduce only one herb at a time, use the lowest possible dose, and track your dog's physical and behavioral responses daily for at least a week.

By staying alert to herbal contraindications and red flags, and by making choices rooted in observation and information rather than assumptions, you help create a safer and more effective path toward natural healing for your dog. This vigilance supports long-term wellness and builds confidence in navigating the dynamic world of canine herbal care.

When to Use Herbs at Home and When to Call the Vet—Decision Checklists

One of the most empowering aspects of using herbal remedies for pets is the ability to take proactive steps toward supporting their health naturally. However, discerning when it's appropriate to provide home-based herbal care versus when a veterinary consultation is essential can be challenging—even stressful. Many pet owners fear making a mistake, overlooking a serious problem, or risking delay when urgent care is needed. To help navigate this gray area, decision checklists and simple flowcharts can provide clarity, confidence, and peace of mind.

Let's begin with situations where it's generally safe and appropriate to use herbs at home. Minor conditions and early symptoms that don't pose an immediate threat often respond well to gentle, supportive herbal treatments. Some examples include mild itching or seasonal allergies, low-level anxiety due to temporary changes (such as guests visiting), occasional indigestion or gassiness, and minor wounds or skin irritations that are clean and not worsening.

To guide you through these situations, consider the following "Safe to Treat at Home" checklist:

- Your pet is eating, drinking, and acting mostly normal.

- Symptoms are mild, not worsening rapidly, and not interfering with daily function.

- The problem is familiar, and your pet has responded well to herbal care for this issue before.

- There is no presence of blood, pus, or foul odor.

- Your pet has no known underlying health conditions that may complicate the issue.

- The herbal treatment chosen is appropriate for the species, and you're confident about dose and use.

If you can confidently check all of the above conditions, beginning with gentle herbal support—while closely observing the response—may be a wise and effective choice.

However, certain warning signs should prompt immediate veterinary attention, regardless of your herbal knowledge or past successes. Rapid-onset symptoms, abnormalities that do not respond to treatment, or anything that causes your pet significant distress should always be taken seriously and not dismissed as something herbs alone can fix.

Keep this "Vet Visit Now" checklist in mind:

- Sudden or severe vomiting, diarrhea, or lethargy.

- Blood in stool, vomit, urine, or from any orifice.

- Difficulty breathing, seizures, or collapse.

- Persistent symptoms that worsen or don't improve within 24–48 hours.

- Ingestion of toxic substances (foods, pharmaceuticals, or plants).

- Unresponsive to home herbal treatments, or symptoms recur repeatedly.

- Your instincts tell you something is seriously wrong.

If even one of these boxes is checked, herbal intervention should not delay professional care. Time can be critical in emergencies, and herbal medicine works best when integrated into a care plan—not as a replacement for necessary diagnostics or treatment.

To simplify the decision-making process in the moment, especially during a stressful episode, it can be helpful to refer to a flowchart like this:

Flowchart: Is This an Emergency?

1. Is your pet breathing normally and responsive?

- No → Call your vet or emergency clinic immediately.

- Yes → Proceed to next question.

1. Are symptoms sudden, severe, or worsening rapidly?

- No → Proceed to next question.

- Yes → Call your vet for urgent advice.

1. Is there vomiting, diarrhea, or discomfort lasting more than 24 hours?

- No → May be safe to monitor with herbs.

- Yes → Schedule a vet visit.

1. Is this a recurring issue you've managed successfully with herbs before?

- Yes → Treat cautiously and monitor.

- No → Consider a vet visit to confirm diagnosis.

Even with these tools, there is no shame in choosing to call the vet "just in case." Combining professional support with your herbal regimen isn't an either/or proposition—it's a comprehensive strategy for your animal's wellness.

To illustrate this, consider two real-world examples with the same pet. In one case, a dog experienced mild digestive upset after eating table scraps. The symptoms included soft stool and minor gas, but no vomiting, distress, or lethargy. With the help of slippery elm bark and a bland diet, symptoms resolved within 24 hours. Herbal care at home was appropriate and effective. Contrast this with a few months later when the same dog developed bloody diarrhea and refused food—a clear sign of something more serious. A prompt vet visit revealed a bacterial infection that required prescription treatment. In both cases, having a clear decision-making framework helped the owner take the right course of action quickly.

Regardless of the approach taken, thorough documentation is crucial. Keeping a symptom tracking journal not only helps you evaluate the effectiveness of herbal remedies but also provides your vet with essential context if the condition escalates. Include details such as:

- Date and time symptoms began.

- Specific symptoms and their progression.

- Herbs or supplements given, with dosage and frequency.

- Changes in appetite, behavior, stool, or urine output.

- Response to treatment over time.

When preparing for a veterinary consultation, bring your notes and be ready to share your herbal protocol. Include the names of the herbs, the form (tincture, powder, tea), the dose given, and the frequency of administration. This transparency ensures that your vet has a complete picture and can guide you safely and effectively. Many veterinarians are open to integrating herbal care when the information is presented clearly and responsibly.

In summary, herbs can be powerful allies for minor ailments and supportive care, but they are not substitutes for veterinary expertise. Using decision checklists, flowcharts, and good documentation allows you to make informed, responsible choices—and ensures your pet receives the care they need when they need it. This thoughtful balance between herbal knowledge and professional guidance is the foundation of integrative pet wellness.

Busting the Top 10 Myths About Herbal Remedies for Dogs

Herbal remedies for dogs have surged in popularity as pet owners seek natural alternatives to conventional veterinary care. While the growing interest in holistic and wellness-based approaches is a positive trend, it's also led to a wave of misinformation. With countless blog posts, social media tips, and DIY recipes circulating online, it's more important than ever to separate fact from fiction. Let's take a closer look at ten of the most common myths surrounding herbal remedies for dogs—and bust them with science, expert insight, and real-life experience.

Myth #1: "All natural means all safe."

Just because something is natural doesn't mean it's harmless. Foxglove and mistletoe are natural—but they're also toxic. Herbs like garlic and tea tree oil, though popular in human use, can be dangerous or even deadly to dogs in certain quantities. According to Dr. Jean Dodds, a leading holistic veterinarian, ""Natural should not be a substitute for qualified veterinary advice."" Just as with pharmaceuticals, herbs need to be dosed appropriately and administered with knowledge of a dog's individual health profile.

Myth #2: "Herbs work instantly."

Herbal medicine is rooted in the principles of slow, supportive healing. Unlike synthetic drugs, which often mask symptoms rapidly, herbs work to correct imbalances over time. Many dog owners become frustrated when a calendula salve doesn't produce results overnight or when a chamomile tincture doesn't immediately calm their anxious pup. In reality, most herbal therapies take days or even weeks to show noticeable benefits, depending on the condition being treated.

Myth #3: "If it's safe for people, it's safe for dogs."

This is one of the most dangerous misconceptions. Dogs metabolize substances differently than humans, and many compounds that are perfectly safe for us can cause serious harm to them. Take xylitol, cocoa, or even essential oils like peppermint—none of which are toxic to humans but can be unsafe for pets. Herbs like St. John's Wort, which can interact with conventional medications in people, can also interfere with veterinary prescriptions in dogs. Always consult a veterinarian familiar with integrative medicine before sharing your human wellness products.

Myth #4: "Online advice is all you need."

Scrolling through forums or social media pages, it's easy to find one-size-fits-all recipes for everything from flea repellents to liver detoxes. A quick image search might even show formula cards encouraging dosages by dog weight—often with little to no scientific backing. One particularly misleading viral post suggested using large doses of turmeric to treat canine arthritis, which resulted in one pet owner's Labrador experiencing severe gastrointestinal upset. Herbal care requires nuance, and online opinions rarely account for breed, age, pre-existing conditions, or interactions with medications.

Myth #5: "Dosage doesn't matter with herbs."

The "a little more won't hurt" mindset is especially harmful in herbal care. Effective dosing isn't just about avoiding toxicity—it's also about ensuring the remedy has the opportunity to work. Too little may be ineffective, too much potentially harmful. Veterinary herbalists stress the importance of calculating safe ranges based on body weight and formulation type, a process that varies between a tea, tincture, or capsule.

Myth #6: "Herbs cure everything."

While herbs offer powerful support, they are not magic bullets. For example, milk thistle can support liver health during recovery from toxins, but it won't reverse permanent liver damage. Valerian root may ease mild anxiety but won't address extreme behavioral disorders or neurological issues. Relying solely on herbs in place of diagnostics and professional advice can delay critical treatment and worsen health outcomes.

Myth #7: "Herbal products labeled 'for dogs' are always trustworthy."

It's alarming, but not surprising: many products marketed as ""all-natural dog supplements"" are poorly regulated. Some contain ineffective doses, questionable ingredients, or misleading health claims. In one product analysis conducted by an independent lab, a popular calming chew was found to contain only 10% of the advertised active ingredients. Look for products backed by third-party testing or those recommended by veterinary professionals.

Myth #8: "A single recipe works for all dogs."

No two dogs are the same. Breed, size, temperament, medical history, and even gut microbiome variations can influence how a dog responds to a remedy. A herb that helps your neighbor's bulldog relieve seasonal allergies might not have the same effect—or could worsen symptoms—in your Pomeranian with food sensitivities. Dog owners must approach herbal remedies with an individualized plan that considers their pet's unique needs.

Myth #9: "Testimonials always prove effectiveness."

While testimonials can be inspirational, they shouldn't replace clinical data. A well-meaning friend's success story using ashwagandha chews might not convey the full picture. In fact, some testimonials cherry-pick positive results while ignoring adverse effects or confounding variables such as concurrent medications. Favor evidence-based sources and consult veterinarians trained in herbal medicine for reliable guidance.

Myth #10: "You don't need to talk to your vet about herbal remedies."

Sadly, this myth persists out of fear: many owners worry that their vets will dismiss natural options off-hand. But keeping your veterinarian in the loop is not only wise—it's vital. Even if your vet isn't versed in herbal therapies, they need to know everything your dog is taking to detect possible interactions or adjust treatment plans accordingly. Integrative veterinarians, who blend conventional and natural approaches, are invaluable resources in safely incorporating herbs into your dog's health regimen.

One illustrative account comes from Sara M., a dog owner in Vermont, who tried an online-recommended "miracle turmeric and black pepper blend" to treat her senior dog's joint pain. When the concoction caused vomiting and discomfort, she turned to a certified veterinary herbalist, who advised gradual introduction with adjusted dosing and liver support herbs. Within six weeks on a personalized protocol, her dog was moving more comfortably—without side effects.

To navigate the maze of herbal claims, pet owners need effective tools. Be on the lookout for vague or absolute terminology like "guaranteed cure" or "safe for all breeds." Cross-reference advice with trusted, science-backed sources such as the American Holistic Veterinary Medical Association (AHVMA), Veterinary Botanical Medicine Association (VBMA), or peer-reviewed veterinary journals.

Before introducing any remedy, use a critical thinking checklist:

- Is the source credible and qualified?
- Is the dosage precisely outlined by weight and species?
- Are there cited studies or veterinary endorsements?
- Is individualized guidance recommended rather than blanket advice?

As herbal medicine becomes more mainstream in canine care, discernment is key. Challenging misinformation and seeking credible, tailored approaches can keep our dogs safe and help them truly benefit from the best of natural healing.

Building Trust—How to Talk to Your Vet About Herbal Protocols

Communicating with your veterinarian about herbal remedies can feel intimidating—especially if you're concerned your approach will be dismissed or misunderstood. Yet, transparency and collaboration are critical to your dog's holistic health. Whether your vet is conventional, integrative, or fully holistic, building trust is the key to productive conversations about herbal care.

For many dog owners just beginning to explore herbal protocols, discomfort often stems from not knowing how to bring up the topic, especially with vets who may not advertise an affinity for natural medicine. If you're feeling anxious, a simple conversation starter can make all the difference. Try: "I've been exploring some gentle herbal support options for my dog's [specific condition, e.g., anxiety or joint stiffness], and I'd love your input." This opens the door without implying that you're trying to replace your vet's medical expertise.

If a vet responds with curiosity or support, great—keep that relationship open and collaborative. If the response is more cautious, remember that skepticism isn't necessarily rejection. Many conventional vets have limited exposure to herbal medicine in their training, and framing the discussion with mutual respect can help pave the way. Try follow-ups like, "I've been using [herb name], and I want to make sure it doesn't interact with any of the medications you're prescribing," or "Have you had other clients use this approach? I'd be interested in your perspective."

One common fear is being judged or brushed off by a vet when disclosing herbal use. This fear is valid—some pet owners have had negative experiences—but hiding herbal supplementation can do more harm than good. Full transparency is essential. Bringing the labels of your herbal products to appointments and offering a typed summary of what you're giving, how much, and for how long, demonstrates that you're organized, informed, and respectful of veterinary input. Many vets find this approach encouraging and professional.

To support this, keeping a Herbal Care Summary is invaluable. Create a simple table that includes columns for the herb name, brand/source, dosage, administration frequency, and any observed effects (e.g., "less itching," or "increased energy"). Print out a copy for your vet and keep one at home as part of your dog's wellness record. This documentation helps your vet evaluate potential herb-drug interactions and ensures everyone on your dog's care team is on the same page.

For those interested in working with a more herb-friendly professional, finding a holistic or integrative vet can be a game changer. Start with directories like the American Holistic Veterinary Medical Association (AHVMA) or the College of Integrative Veterinary Therapies. When interviewing new vets, ask questions like: "What's your experience with herbal medicine?" or "Are you open to partnering with a herbalist or using botanical treatments alongside conventional care?" The goal is to find someone who takes a balanced approach, appreciates your involvement, and is willing to learn with you if needed.

Real-life stories underscore how powerful vet-owner partnerships can be when both sides communicate openly. One owner of a senior Labrador with arthritis shared how their conventional vet initially had no experience with devil's claw or boswellia, but after reviewing the summary and label information, agreed to monitor its effects as part of a broader management plan. The result? Improved mobility, reduced NSAID dosage, and a more collaborative vet-client relationship than ever before.

At the heart of these conversations is a mutual goal—your dog's well-being. So when visiting the vet, keep a few basic dos and don'ts in mind. Do be honest about every supplement or herb you're administering. Do bring the actual product or its label. Don't become defensive if a vet expresses concerns—listen, ask questions, and be ready to find common ground. Most importantly, remember that both herbalists and veterinarians bring something valuable to the table.

When you communicate clearly, document thoughtfully, and approach your vet with respect and openness, you become not just your dog's caregiver but their advocate. In doing so, you lay the foundation for a team-based approach that honors both traditional medicine and nature's wisdom—ensuring your dog benefits from the best of both worlds.

Getting Started—Your Herbal Toolkit and Sourcing Essentials

For centuries, humans have turned to the healing power of plants—and our dogs can benefit from this same wisdom. Canine herbalism isn't about replacing your vet or ignoring modern medicine; it's about working with nature to support your dog's health, prevent problems before they start, and give their body the tools it needs to heal itself. When used thoughtfully, herbs can be powerful allies for everything from boosting immunity to easing joint discomfort, supporting digestion, and even calming anxiety.

In this chapter, we'll lay the groundwork for understanding what canine herbalism is (and isn't), how it works within your dog's unique biology, and why a holistic approach looks at the whole animal—not just isolated symptoms. We'll explore the different categories of herbs, the roles they play, and how to start thinking about your dog's wellness in a way that blends traditional knowledge with modern veterinary insight.

By the end, you'll have a clear picture of how herbs fit into a balanced care plan for your dog, along with the confidence to begin using them safely, effectively, and in harmony with your dog's overall health needs.

Essential Starter Herbs Every Dog Parent Should Have

When it comes to natural wellness for dogs, certain herbs stand out not only for their gentle efficacy but also for their versatility and ease of use. Whether you're supporting your dog's digestion, calming their nerves, or caring for their skin, a thoughtfully chosen herbal toolkit can become a powerful ally in holistic pet care. Below is a curated selection of must-have starter herbs—ideal for beginners—chosen for their safety, multi-purpose applications, and availability in most health stores or online marketplaces.

Chamomile is perhaps the most well-known calming herb, gentle enough for dogs yet effective across multiple issues. Its soothing properties make it a go-to for easing anxiety, settling an upset stomach, and calming skin irritations when applied topically. Whether brewed as a tea or infused in oil for a salve, chamomile is a staple in any herbal first-aid kit.

Chamomile - fresh, dried, and packaged

Calendula, with its brilliant orange-yellow blossoms, offers exceptional support for wounds, skin irritations, and fungal infections. Its antiseptic and anti-inflammatory qualities make it ideal for creating healing salves or gentle rinses for minor cuts and hot spots. Calendula is typically used topically but can also be made into a mild tea for internal soothing.

Calendula - fresh blossoms, dried petals, and calendula salve

Ginger is not only a culinary delight but an invaluable herb for dogs dealing with nausea, motion sickness, or digestive sluggishness. In small, appropriate doses, fresh or powdered ginger can help relieve gas, stimulate appetite, and support immune health. It's particularly helpful for dogs who get carsick during travel.

Ginger - raw root, powdered form, and capsule supplement

Peppermint, thanks to its cooling menthol content, works well for mild digestive disturbances, such as bloating and indigestion. Though potent, when used sparingly and correctly (preferably as a weak tea), peppermint can provide gentle relief and freshen a dog's breath. Avoid concentrated essential oils, which are too strong for internal canine use.

Peppermint - fresh leaves, dried tea, and packaged dog-safe tea blend

Marshmallow Root, a mucilaginous herb, is deeply soothing to inflamed mucous membranes in the gastrointestinal and urinary tracts. Its slippery texture helps ease coughing, acid reflux, UTIs, and general stomach upset. Whether given as a cold infusion or mixed with food, marshmallow root is a gentle support with wide-reaching effects.

Marshmallow Root - dried root pieces, powdered extract, and rehydrated cold infusion

Turmeric is renowned for its anti-inflammatory effects, especially beneficial for dogs with arthritis or joint stiffness. Rich in curcumin, turmeric also offers antioxidant and liver-supportive benefits. Combined with a small amount of black pepper and healthy fat, it becomes more bioavailable and effective, often provided as ""golden paste.""

Turmeric - fresh root, powdered spice, and golden paste in jar

Slippery Elm is a gut-friendly herb that coats and protects the digestive tract, making it ideal for diarrhea, vomiting, or upset stomach. It's often used during episodes of GI distress in both acute and chronic cases. Only use sustainably harvested slippery elm to ensure environmental responsibility.

Slippery Elm - powdered form, capsules, and prepared gruel

Each of these herbs earns its place not just for one-purpose use, but for their flexibility. Chamomile, for example, helps both anxious behavior and itchy skin; peppermint not only soothes the gut but also works as a mild insect deterrent; turmeric supports joints and bolsters immune function. Moreover, these herbs are generally safe when used correctly and easy to find in natural food stores, pet specialty shops, or reputable herbal suppliers.

To help you get started, here's a quick-reference chart highlighting core uses, basic dose ranges, and key safety tips:

Herb	Key Uses	Basic Dosage*	Safety Notes
Chamomile	Anxiety, skin irritation, digestive upset	1/4 tsp dried flower per 20 lbs (tea)	Avoid if allergic to ragweed
Calendula	Wounds, hot spots, ear infections	Topical use or tea rinse	Safe topically, minimal internal use
Ginger	Motion sickness, nausea, digestion	Small pinch per 10 lbs (powder)	Use caution with bleeding disorders
Peppermint	Gas, bloating, mild nausea	Weak tea, 1–2 tsp per 20 lbs	Avoid essential oil form internally
Marshmallow Root	UTIs, acid reflux, throat irritation	1/4 tsp dried root per 20 lbs (tea)	Can reduce absorption of medications
Turmeric	Inflammation, joint support, liver health	1/8–1/4 tsp per 10 lbs (with fat/pepper)	Monitor for constipation or GI upset
Slippery Elm	Diarrhea, vomiting, GI inflammation	1/4 tsp powder mixed with water per 10 lbs	Use sustainably harvested only

*Always consult with your veterinarian before introducing herbs, especially if your dog is on medication or has a health condition.

These foundational herbs create a well-rounded, natural health cabinet for dog parents seeking gentle, effective solutions. By starting with this essential set, you'll be well-equipped to support your dog's wellness journey safely and knowledgeably. In the next section, we'll explore how to prepare and store these herbs properly to maximize their benefits and shelf life.

Where to Buy High-Quality, Dog-Safe Herbs—Online and Local Resources

Finding high-quality, dog-safe herbs requires more than just selecting the prettiest packaging or clicking on the first online listing. When your pet's health is at stake, sourcing herbs with safety, freshness, and purity in mind is essential. Thankfully, there are a variety of trustworthy options to secure herbs that meet these standards, both online and locally.

For online shoppers, several reputable herbal retailers stand out for their commitment to quality and transparency. Mountain Rose Herbs and Starwest Botanicals are frequently recommended for their organic and sustainably harvested selections, along with detailed sourcing information on each product. These companies often carry certifications such as USDA Organic or Non-GMO Project Verified, giving pet parents peace of mind. Additionally, Etsy can be a surprisingly rich source as long as you choose sellers who provide clear information about their ingredients, cleanliness, and practices. Look for shops with reviews that specifically mention pet use, and prioritize sellers who indicate their products are safe for canine consumption or who possess credentials in herbalism or veterinary herbal applications.

Those who prefer to shop in-person can often find excellent options at their local health food store or independent herb shop. These boutiques usually employ knowledgeable staff who can guide you toward dog-safe selections and even suggest preparation methods for home use. Pet boutiques that specialize in holistic or natural products may also carry ready-to-use herbal items crafted especially for dogs, labeled with clear dosing and usage instructions.

Before making a purchase—whether online or in-store—it's important to vet any new supplier carefully. Begin by checking if they provide full transparency about sourcing, including country of origin, organic or wildcrafted status, and any third-party testing. Suppliers who certify their herbs as pesticide-free or free from irradiation are ideal. Don't hesitate to reach out and ask questions like: Are these herbs suitable for pets? How are they processed and packaged? Are there any additives?

A "Supplier Vetting Checklist" might include looking for labels such as USDA Organic, Certified Naturally Grown, or FairWild-certified. Be cautious of brands that use vague language like "natural" without qualification, or those that refuse to disclose sourcing information. Also, avoid herbs sold in mixed blends unless specifically formulated for dogs, as many blends intended for human use contain ingredients harmful to pets—like garlic, cocoa shells, or essential oils.

Buying in bulk may be tempting, but for household use it's usually best to stick to small quantities to ensure freshness. Dried herbs, when stored properly, retain potency for up to a year. Purchasing just what you need reduces waste and keeps your dog's remedies effective. Budget-conscious buyers might consider community bulk-buys or CO-OPs, where herbs are purchased in larger quantities and distributed among members—this approach can significantly cut costs while maintaining quality.

For those in areas where specialty resources aren't available, more accessible options do exist. Supermarkets increasingly carry basic herbs like chamomile, rosemary, and peppermint in their spice sections, which can be safe for dogs if purchased in pure, unsweetened forms. On Amazon, some trusted brands offer high-quality single-herb powders or dried forms with clear sourcing information and ingredient purity. Look for companies that publish lab results or ingredient sourcing details in their product descriptions. However, shoppers should be wary of herb blends or capsules sold for human wellness, as these often contain fillers, sweeteners, or potentially toxic add-ons unsafe for canine consumption.

In the end, responsible sourcing is the foundation of safely using herbs for your dog. Whether you're shopping online, supporting a local store, or piecing together safe options from a supermarket shelf, your diligence in selecting fresh, properly labeled herbs will directly contribute to your pet's wellbeing. As we move forward, we'll explore how to properly store and prepare these herbs to ensure their healing potential remains intact.

Urban Foraging and Small-Space Herb Growing for Beginners

Growing your own herbs and foraging in urban environments are both rewarding and surprisingly accessible, even for beginners living in small apartments or city dwellings. With a little creativity and knowledge, anyone can cultivate a thriving mini-garden on a windowsill or discover edible and medicinal plants in nearby parks and alleys. Whether you're hoping to start a calming tea garden or simply want to learn how to responsibly gather herbs from the urban landscape, this guide has you covered with practical guidance tailored for limited spaces and city life.

For beginners looking to grow herbs at home, calendula, peppermint, and chamomile are ideal starter choices. They are not only forgiving to novice gardeners but also highly useful for culinary and medicinal purposes. First, choose suitable containers with good drainage—recycled pots, ceramic planters, or even plastic tubs work well as long as they have holes at the bottom. Calendula prefers shallow containers (at least 6 inches deep), while peppermint and chamomile benefit from slightly deeper pots (8–10 inches).

Position your containers in spots that receive at least 4–6 hours of sunlight daily. Windowsills facing south or west are often ideal, while balconies and patios can support more robust growth. Calendula thrives in full sun with well-draining, loamy soil. Peppermint is hardy and prefers partial shade and moist, rich soil, while chamomile grows best in slightly sandy, moderately moist soil conditions. Overwatering is one of the most common mistakes—allow the top one inch of soil to dry out between watering, especially with peppermint and chamomile, which can rot in soggy conditions.

Beyond container gardening, urban foraging offers a fascinating way to connect with local flora and supplement your herb collection. The key to safe foraging is identification and awareness. Always positively identify a plant before harvesting—mistaking a toxic species for an edible one can have serious consequences. Use reputable field guides and foraging apps to learn distinguishing features, and seek out well-known ""starter"" herbs like dandelion, plantain, and lamb's quarters, which are abundant and relatively easy to recognize.

A basic foraging safety checklist includes: knowing the plant's identity for certain, avoiding harvests from roadsides or areas likely sprayed with pesticides, harvesting sparingly to promote regrowth, and following local laws. Many cities have regulations about foraging in public parks; while some municipalities permit light foraging of invasive or non-listed species, others strictly prohibit it. Always research your local guidelines before picking anything. Look for urban green spots maintained without herbicides and avoid areas near traffic, pet relief zones, or industrial runoff.

City gardening poses unique challenges, but these can be addressed with simple, effective solutions. One common issue is limited sunlight—many urban dwellers only have access to shaded windows or covered balconies. To ensure healthy herb growth, consider rotating your containers to chase the sun or supplement low-light settings with inexpensive grow lights. If you have curious pets that love to dig, try pet-proofing your planters with chicken wire lids, placing citrus peels around the soil, or elevating containers to out-of-reach shelves.

Pests might also show up indoors or in balcony gardens, especially aphids and whiteflies. A natural and aesthetic solution is companion planting—placing herbs that repel pests together. For instance, placing garlic or basil near chamomile helps deter aphids, while planting mint near calendula can prevent spider mites from settling in.

To guide you visually, it's helpful to know how healthy herb plants should look. Calendula should have upright stems and bright yellow-orange blooms with no leaf curling. Healthy peppermint has dark green, aromatic leaves with no wilting or brown edges, and chamomile should maintain delicate white flowers and feathery foliage that doesn't appear dry or brittle. If your plant droops, yellows, or wilts despite regular care, check your watering habits and review soil drainage.

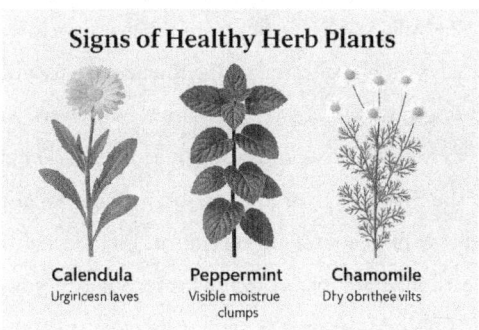

Signs of Healthy Herb Plants

Calendula — Urgiricesn laves
Peppermint — Visible moistrue clumps
Chamomile — Dry obrithee vilts

Once your herbs mature, harvesting them is simple. Snip leaves and blooms with clean scissors in the morning after the dew has dried but before the sun is at its peak, when essential oils are most concentrated. To dry herbs for later use, bundle and hang them upside-down in a cool, dry place away from direct sunlight. Alternatively, a mesh drying rack indoors works beautifully for petals like calendula or chamomile.

Urban foraging and small-space herb growing are accessible, empowering practices that connect us with nature even in the heart of the city. With a few containers, some sunlight, and curiosity about your local environment, you can begin cultivating and harvesting herbs with confidence and care. Up next, we'll explore how to incorporate your homegrown or foraged herbs into practical preparations like teas, salves, and tinctures."

Reading Herb Labels—Spotting Additives, Fillers, and Red Flags

Selecting high-quality herbs means going beyond just checking the name on the front of the package—it requires learning how to read and interpret ingredient labels thoroughly. Whether you're buying dried herbs in bulk, fresh bundles from the grocery store, or supplements labeled with herbal extracts, the fine print tells a deeper story. Understanding how to decode these labels empowers you to avoid unnecessary additives, fillers, and even misleading marketing language.

One of the first things to look for on an herb label is the presence of additives or fillers. Common culprits include maltodextrin—a processed carbohydrate that's often used to bulk up powders or improve shelf stability—as well as artificial flavors, silicon dioxide, or synthetic preservatives like sodium benzoate. While these ingredients might serve a functional purpose in mass manufacturing, they can dilute the purity and effectiveness of the herb, and in some cases, cause adverse reactions, especially for sensitive individuals or pets.

Also be mindful of vague or overly complex ingredient lists. When an herb or blend contains more than just the listed botanical, each additional component should be clearly named. For example, a dried basil product shouldn't include anything but basil leaves. If you see "natural flavors" or "color added," dig deeper—they may be hiding chemical compounds not immediately apparent. Be especially cautious with supplement herbs marketed as capsules or powders. Many of these include binding agents, flow enhancers like magnesium stearate, or coatings not listed clearly.

An area that deserves particular scrutiny is the terminology "proprietary blend." This phrase, while common on supplement bottles, should serve as a red flag. It allows manufacturers to list a group of ingredients without revealing the quantity of each one. For instance, a label that lists a "digestive support blend (turmeric, ginger, fennel)" may contain mostly one inexpensive ingredient, with only trace amounts of the others. Since potency is often dosage-dependent, these blends can be misleading in terms of their therapeutic value.

Different types of herb products—culinary, supplemental, and pet-specific—are each subject to distinct labeling regulations, which can make comparison difficult. Culinary herbs, which fall under food labeling laws, must list all ingredients but often aren't required to disclose origins unless marked organic. Supplemental herbs, regulated differently as dietary supplements by authorities like the FDA in the U.S., often have looser requirements and can legally include non-active fillers if listed somewhere on the label. Pet supplements, meanwhile, fall into a less regulated gray area depending on whether they are labeled as food, medicine, or treats, which can mean even less transparency. For pet owners especially, this inconsistency can pose risks when additives are not disclosed or tested for safety in animals.

It's also easy to be swayed by marketing claims like "100% natural," "eco-friendly," or "doctor-recommended," which aren't always backed by regulatory standards. To cut through the hype, seek out labels that include third-party certification logos such as USDA Organic, Non-GMO Project Verified, or NSF Certified. These endorsements require products to meet certain verification steps that enhance credibility. Some high-quality brands also include QR codes on their labels that link to lab testing results or Certificates of Analysis (COAs), providing transparency about purity, potency, and contaminant testing—a practice that's becoming more common in reputable herbal products.

In a marketplace flooded with options, strong label literacy helps consumers distinguish between reputable, high-quality herbs and those merely masked in fine print and flashy marketing. Armed with this knowledge, you'll be better equipped to choose herbs that are potent, safe, and ethically produced—whether you're cooking a flavorful dish, supplementing your wellness regimen, or caring for a furry companion.

Herb Storage, Shelf Life, and Spoilage

Proper storage of herbs is essential to preserving their potency, flavor, and safety—especially when it comes to using them in homemade remedies or pet care formulations. Whether dried, powdered, or in tincture form, herbs are highly sensitive to environmental conditions. Storing them correctly can mean the difference between an effective natural remedy and a risky or ineffective one.

The best containers for herb storage are airtight, light-resistant, and non-reactive. Glass jars with tight-fitting lids are commonly used because they don't leach chemicals and allow for easy monitoring of herb condition. Amber or cobalt blue jars, in particular, offer extra protection from ultraviolet light, which can degrade the quality of herbs over time. Metal tins lined with food-safe finishes are another excellent option, as are heavy-duty opaque pouches with resealable closures. Avoid plastic containers whenever possible, as they can retain odors and absorb oils, diminishing both the herb's freshness and shelf life.

Herbs should be stored in a cool, dry location away from direct sunlight and sources of heat or humidity—kitchen cupboards, high shelves near ovens, or sunny countertops are all poor choices. Instead, opt for a dark pantry, a storage drawer, or a designated herb cabinet. Moisture is one of the most common culprits behind spoilage and mold growth, so it's important to never open storage containers in steam-filled areas like bathrooms or kitchens. Always use dry, clean utensils when handling herbs to avoid introducing contaminants.

Recognizing when an herb has passed its prime is a key skill. When evaluating the condition of herbs, visual and sensory cues are your guide. Fresh dried herbs should retain a vibrant color reflective of their original form—bright green for mint, basil, or parsley, deep orange for turmeric, or rich browns for cinnamon and root barks. Faded, yellowed, or grayish tones often indicate the herb has oxidized and lost its potency. Aroma is equally critical; herbs should have a strong, distinctive scent. If the smell is faint, musty, or sour, it's likely the herb has deteriorated. Texture also matters—leaves should be crumbly but not dusty, and roots or barks should snap, not bend. Sliminess, visible mold (white, green, or black fuzz), or webbing are unmistakable signs of spoilage and immediate grounds for disposal.

Visual comparisons can be especially helpful: imagine two jars of dried oregano. In the fresh jar, the leaves are a deep forest green with a strong, clean herbal smell. In the spoiled batch, leaves are pale and crumble into a fine powder with little to no aroma, and on closer inspection, you may spot tiny white specks of mold clinging to the glass. Whenever in doubt, it's best to discard questionable herbs rather than risk using them.

Different herb forms have different shelf lives. A quick-reference guide can simplify tracking their usability:

Herb Form	Typical Shelf Life
Dried Leaves	1 to 2 years
Dried Roots/Barks	2 to 3 years
Powders (e.g., turmeric)	1 year
Tinctures (alcohol-based)	3 to 5 years
Tinctures (glycerin-based)	1 to 2 years
Infused oils	6 to 12 months

Ensure labels include both the herb name and the date of purchase or preparation. A simple DIY labeling system might involve masking tape and a permanent marker, or printable label templates that you update and affix to each jar. For example, a label might read: "Chamomile Flowers – Purchased March 2023 – Use By March 2025." Keep an inventory list so you can rotate stock efficiently, using older herbs first and discarding them when they pass their expiration window.

When disposing of expired or contaminated herbs, do not compost them unless you are certain they are free of mold or pathogens. For safety, especially around pets who may be prone to sniffing and sampling, seal spoiled herbs in a paper bag or biodegradable pouch and place it inside a trash bin with a lid. If discarding liquids like expired tinctures or oils, avoid pouring them down the sink. Instead, soak them into an absorbent material like kitty litter or coffee grounds before placing in the trash.

In conclusion, effectively storing and managing your herb collection not only preserves the healing potential of your botanicals but also ensures the safety of anyone (furry companions included) using them. By understanding the visual and sensory markers of freshness and spoilage and applying thoughtful organization, you can build a safe, potent, and longer-lasting herbal apothecary.

Herbal Preparation Methods—DIY Remedies Made Simple

Nature has long offered a pharmacy of healing plants—wildflowers, barks, roots, and leaves that soothe, restore, and strengthen body and mind. But often, the wisdom of preparing these natural remedies feels cloaked in mystery or outdated tradition. That ends now. In this chapter, we roll up our sleeves and dive into the world of herbal preparation in a way that's deeply practical, grounded in tradition, and yet perfectly suited for your modern kitchen.

Herbal Preparation Methods—DIY Remedies Made Simple empowers you to create your own herbal medicine cabinet using time-tested techniques tailored for beginners and seasoned herbalists alike. We'll explore the essentials of crafting tinctures, teas, salves, oils, syrups, and more—with step-by-step guidance using tools you already have at home. You'll discover how to choose the most effective preparation method for specific herbs and ailments, from calming teas for stress relief to potent immune-boosting tinctures.

We'll also discuss important considerations like proper sourcing, safe dosages, storage, and shelf life, so you can create remedies confidently and responsibly. Each section demystifies the process, combining the wisdom of generations with clear, modern instructions.

Whether you're looking to take control of your wellness routine, reconnect with nature, or simply explore the healing power that grows all around us, this chapter is your gateway. By the time you turn the last page, you won't just know how herbs heal—you'll know exactly how to prepare them, preserve them, and use them with purpose. Let's begin the journey from leaf to life.

Infusions, Decoctions, and Teas—Step-by-Step for Every Dog Size

Herbal teas, infusions, and decoctions are gentle yet powerful ways to support your dog's health naturally. While they may sound similar, understanding how they differ—and when to use each—can ensure that your pup receives the maximum benefit in the safest way possible.

Infusions are best suited for soft plant parts such as leaves and flowers. These are steeped rather than simmered to preserve their delicate properties. A good example of this is chamomile flowers, which are often used in infusions to help reduce anxiety or promote restful sleep for dogs. Simply steeping chamomile in hot water (but not boiling it) allows the compounds to release gently, making it an ideal choice for nervous or high-strung pups.

Decoctions, on the other hand, are meant for the tougher parts of plants, such as roots, bark, and seeds. These require heat and time to extract their beneficial compounds. Ginger root, for example, is commonly used in decoctions to support digestion and reduce nausea. The simmering process helps to draw out the active components that can help soothe an upset stomach or prevent motion sickness in dogs.

Here's how to prepare these remedies based on your dog's size, using ingredients and methods tailored to canine needs. A standard ratio is 1 teaspoon of dried herb or 1 tablespoon of fresh herb per 8 ounces (1 cup) of water. For infusions, simply pour just-boiled water over the herb, cover, and steep for 10–15 minutes. Strain out the herbs and let the liquid cool completely to room temperature before serving it to your dog. For decoctions, add the chopped root or bark to cold water, bring it to a boil, then reduce to a simmer for 20–30 minutes. Strain and cool thoroughly before offering it to your dog.

To accurately tailor doses based on your dog's weight, it's essential to follow serving guidelines. The general rule of thumb is to offer 1 teaspoon of herbal tea per 10 pounds of body weight, up to a tablespoon for larger dogs. For quick reference, here's a simplified dosage chart:

Dog Size	Weight Range	Serving Amount
Toy	Under 10 lbs	½ to 1 tsp
Small	10–25 lbs	1–2 tsp
Medium	26–50 lbs	1–2 tbsp
Large	51–80 lbs	2–3 tbsp
Giant	Over 80 lbs	¼ cup (4 tbsp)

Always allow the tea to cool completely before offering it. Never serve herbs steeped in hot or even warm liquid, as dogs are especially sensitive to temperature and could burn their mouths or throats.

For pet parents with busy schedules, batch-preparing herbal teas can be a lifesaver. After steeping or simmering, pour cooled teas into ice cube trays and freeze. Once frozen, you can transfer the cubes into labeled freezer bags for easy storage. Each cube can be thawed and added to your dog's water bowl or mixed into food. Cooled teas can also be stored in the refrigerator in sealed jars for up to three days. This not only ensures freshness but allows for seamless integration into your dog's daily routine.

Incorporating herbal teas into your dog's care regimen offers a gentle, effective way to support wellness naturally. Whether you're addressing anxiety, digestion, or general hydration and wellness, understanding these methods allows you to prepare safe and effective remedies—no matter the size of your furry friend. As we move forward, we'll explore specific herbal recipes tailored for common canine conditions.

Making Alcohol-Free Tinctures and Glycerites for Sensitive Dogs

For pet parents looking to support their dog's health naturally, tinctures offer a convenient and effective way to deliver the benefits of herbs. However, standard tinctures are typically made using alcohol—a substance that can be harmful and unpalatable for dogs, especially those with sensitive systems. The good news is that there are dog-safe alternatives: glycerites and alcohol-free tinctures, which use vegetable glycerin as the primary solvent instead of alcohol.

Vegetable glycerin is a clear, slightly sweet, syrup-like liquid derived from plant oils such as coconut or palm. Unlike alcohol, it's non-toxic, gentle on the digestive system, and actually pleasant in taste—making it particularly suitable for pets. In herbal preparations, glycerin still acts as a solvent that extracts medicinal compounds from plants, though it may not draw out some constituents as powerfully as alcohol does. Nevertheless, for many of the herbs commonly used in canine care, glycerin is an ideal, safe, and reliable medium.

Creating alcohol-free tinctures at home is a rewarding process requiring minimal equipment and no prior experience. To start, choose the dried herb best suited for your dog's needs—such as chamomile for anxiety or marshmallow root for digestive support. You'll need a clean glass mason jar, dried herbs, food-grade vegetable glycerin (make sure it's 100% pure and not mixed with alcohol), and filtered water. For a standard recipe, combine one part dried herbs to five parts liquid, with the liquid being made up of 60% vegetable glycerin and 40% water. For example, if you're using 1 cup of dried herb, you would mix 3 cups of glycerin with 2 cups of filtered water.

Place the herbs in the jar and pour the glycerin-water mixture over them, ensuring the herbs are fully submerged. Stir or shake gently, then seal the jar with a tight-fitting lid. Label the jar with the date and the contents. Store it in a cool, dark location for 2 to 4 weeks, shaking it daily to maximize extraction. After this infusion period, strain the liquid through a fine mesh sieve or cheesecloth into a clean bowl or container. Squeeze or press the herbs to retrieve as much liquid as possible. Finally, transfer the completed glycerite into amber glass dropper bottles to protect it from light and maintain its potency.

Shelf life for homemade glycerites is typically around one year when stored in a cool, dark place away from direct sunlight. Always label each bottle with the herbal ingredients, date prepared, and recommended purpose. If any smell, color, or texture changes occur, it's best to discard the tincture and make a fresh batch.

Once you've prepared your dog-safe tincture, administration becomes the next important step. Dosage depends on both the specific herb and your dog's weight. As a general guideline, a typical dosage may range from 1/4 teaspoon for small dogs (under 20 lbs), 1/2 teaspoon for medium dogs (20–50 lbs), to 1 teaspoon for large dogs (over 50 lbs), up to twice daily. Always consult your veterinarian, preferably one experienced with herbal medicine, before starting any new supplement regimen.

For particularly picky or suspicious dogs, you can disguise the taste of the tincture by mixing it into moist food, dog-safe yogurt, broth, or even a thin layer of natural, xylitol-free peanut butter. Some dogs tolerate it well directly from a dropper, especially if gently placed into the side of the mouth rather than on the tongue to avoid startling them.

Crafting your own alcohol-free tinctures allows you to support your dog's well-being with natural, customized remedies. By understanding how to make and store glycerites safely, you can offer gentle, effective care—tailored specifically for your four-legged companion.

DIY Salves and Balms—Batch-Prep for Itchy Skin and Minor Wounds

Creating your own herbal salves and balms at home is a rewarding and cost-effective way to support your dog's skin health using natural, dog-safe ingredients. Whether you're addressing minor cuts, dry patches, or seasonal itchiness, a well-crafted salve can soothe irritation and protect delicate skin. By batch-prepping a few basic recipes with multi-purpose properties, you'll always have a ready supply on hand when your canine companion needs it.

The foundation of most homemade salves starts with a dog-safe carrier oil such as olive oil, which is gentle and deeply moisturizing. Infusing this oil with healing herbs like calendula and chamomile adds powerful skin-soothing properties. To make an herbal-infused oil, place about 1 cup of dried calendula flowers and chamomile blossoms in a clean, dry glass jar and cover them fully with 1.5 cups of olive oil. Seal the jar and let it steep in a warm, sunny spot for 2–3 weeks, shaking it gently every day, or use a quick method by gently warming the herbs in the oil over a double boiler for 1–2 hours—never letting the oil exceed 120°F (49°C) for optimal preservation of the plant benefits.

Once your herbal oil is ready, strain the herbs through cheesecloth or a fine mesh sieve into a clean measuring cup. Combine the infused oil with beeswax to form the salve—approximately 1 ounce (by weight) of beeswax to every 4 ounces (by volume) of oil will give you a firm but spreadable consistency. Using a double boiler, melt the beeswax first, then add the infused oil and stir continually until fully blended. Testing the consistency is easy: drip a small spoonful onto a cool plate and let it harden—it should be firm but allow your finger to press into it without much resistance. Adjust by adding more beeswax for a firmer balm, or more oil for a softer one.

Pour the slightly cooled (but still pourable) mixture into clean, dry tins or glass jars. Label each container with the date and ingredients used. Store at room temperature in a cool, dry place for up to 6–12 months. Adding a few drops of vitamin E oil per jar can also act as a natural preservative while giving an extra boost to skin repair.

Customizing your salves for specific uses is simple and allows you to tailor care to your dog's needs. For calming itchy or irritated skin, a few drops of lavender essential oil (ensure it's high-quality and used at safe dilution: no more than 1–2 drops per 4 oz batch) can be soothing without overwhelming a dog's sensitive nose. Marshmallow root, known for its mucilaginous and cooling effects, can be added to the infusion to further alleviate inflammation or reactions to bug bites or grass allergies. For a nourishing paw balm, blend in shea butter or coconut oil for elasticity and extra moisture.

When it comes to application, always clean the area gently with warm water and pat dry before applying a salve. Use clean fingers or a dedicated spatula and apply a thin layer. Since dogs often lick freshly treated areas, use distraction techniques such as chew treats or apply just before a walk. Dog booties can be helpful to protect paws after applying balm, preventing ingestion and preserving the effects.

Homemade salves and balms bring peace of mind—you know exactly what ingredients are being used, and you can tailor each batch for your dog's unique skin sensitivities. With a few thoughtful ingredients and some simple tools, you can create a reliable herbal toolkit for handling everything from itchy hotspots to dry paw pads. In the next section, we'll explore natural sprays and cleansers to round out your canine skin care arsenal.

Powders, Capsules, and Treats—Palatable Options for Picky Pups

For dog owners exploring herbal remedies, the biggest challenge often isn't selecting the right herb—but getting a picky pup to ingest it. Fortunately, with a little creativity, it's entirely possible to incorporate beneficial herbs into your dog's routine through palatable and easy-to-administer options like powders, capsules, and tasty treats. These methods not only make herbal supplementation more enjoyable for your dog but also simplify portion control and dosing.

Turning dried herbs into usable powders starts with the proper preparation. Once you've sourced dog-safe herbs—such as chamomile, dandelion root, or ginger—the next step is grinding. Using a standard coffee or spice grinder, dried leaves, roots, or seeds can be pulverized into a fine powder for easier mixing, measuring, and storage. These powders can then be dispensed in a number of ways depending on your dog's preferences.

One of the most convenient methods is filling gelatin capsules with pre-measured doses. Empty gelatin or vegan capsules (usually size '0' or '00' are ideal for dogs, depending on your dog's weight and dosage requirement) are readily available online or in natural health stores. To fill them, use a capsule-filling tray or, for small batches, simply scoop the powdered herb into each half of the capsule by hand. This allows you to create individualized, mess-free herbal supplements that can be hidden in food or given like a treat.

For pups who refuse capsules or those who can detect even the faintest herbal aroma, creating dog-approved herbal treats is often the secret weapon. Homemade recipes can help mask strong or unfamiliar tastes, transforming medication time into treat time. A foolproof favorite is the peanut butter and pumpkin ""herbal treat ball."" Using unsweetened canned pumpkin, natural peanut butter (xylitol-free), and a binding grain like oat flour, you can mix in a precise dose of powdered herbs before shaping small bite-sized balls and refrigerating them.

Another excellent option for warm weather or teething pups involves frozen yogurt-herb cubes. By blending plain, unsweetened yogurt with your chosen herbal powder and optional flavor enhancers—like mashed banana or bone broth—you can pour the mixture into silicone molds or ice cube trays. Once frozen, these become cooling, medicinal snacks that serve as a practical herbal delivery method.

To ensure the longevity and effectiveness of your homemade supplements, proper storage is key. Herbal powders should be stored in airtight, dark-colored glass jars in a cool, dark cupboard to maintain potency. Treats, both baked and frozen, should be kept in freezer-safe containers or bags. Treat balls generally last a week in the refrigerator or up to three months in the freezer, while herb-infused yogurt cubes can be stored frozen for similar durations.

Even with the tastiest recipes, some dogs remain skeptical. For these extra-picky pups, consider mixing herbs or capsules into a small amount of their favorite wet food, bone broth, or even a spoonful of tuna or sardine juice. These strongly flavored additions can overpower even the most bitter herbal taste and entice dogs who otherwise shy away from new foods. Another trick is to warm the food slightly (never hot), which enhances the aroma and appeal.

Incorporating herbs into your dog's diet doesn't have to be a battle. With the right mixing methods, tasty delivery systems, and a bit of clever masking, even the most selective eaters can be coaxed into embracing herbal support. By blending nutrition with flavor, you're not just helping your pup feel better—you're making the experience enjoyable for both of you.

Finished Remedy Photo Gallery—What Your DIY Should Look Like

When making your own herbal remedies at home, visual cues can be just as important as written instructions. Whether you're steeping a tea, bottling a tincture, or whipping up a salve, knowing exactly what your finished product should look like boosts both your confidence and the safety of your creations. This finished remedy photo gallery serves as a visual guide to help you recognize when a remedy is successful—and when it might need a do-over.

Let's start with herbal teas. A well-made infusion or decoction should be vibrant, with colors ranging from pale yellow to deep amber or even dark brown, depending on the herbs used. A high-quality tea is usually translucent but not necessarily crystal clear. If your tea is cloudy due to fine sediment, that's generally fine—especially with powdered herbs—but if it appears murky or has a slimy texture, it could indicate spoilage or contamination. Side-by-side photos in this section illustrate the difference between a clean, steeped herbal tea and one that has become overly steeped or improperly stored.

Tinctures are another common DIY remedy, often stored in amber dropper bottles for preservation. A successful tincture will typically have a rich color that reflects the herb—think golden from chamomile or dark green from nettle—and minimal sediment. Clear labeling is critical; the gallery shows examples of perfectly labeled tinctures with dates, herb names, and alcohol ratios. We also explore how the right bottle lightproofing and seal ensure shelf stability.

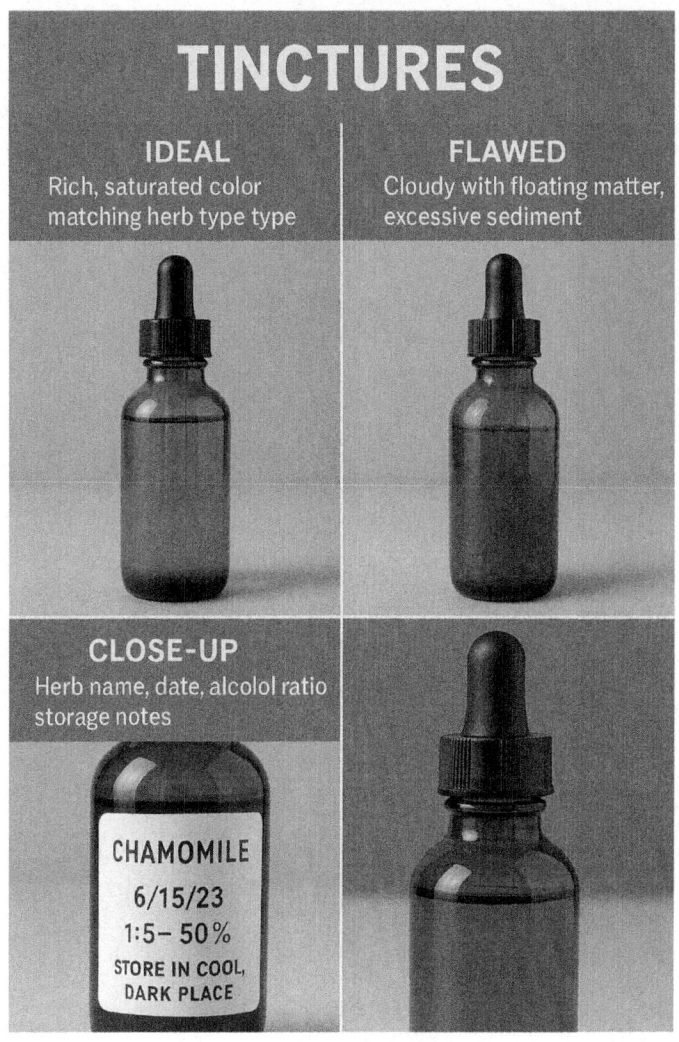

For salves and balms, visual texture and consistency are key indicators of quality. A fresh finished salve should be smooth and uniform in color, without noticeable graininess, separation, or mold growth. Spoiled salves may develop white or fuzzy patches, or separate into oily and waxy layers. To build your discernment, we offer side-by-side photos comparing a perfectly emulsified calendula salve next to one that has separated or gone rancid—noting what went wrong and how to fix it next time.

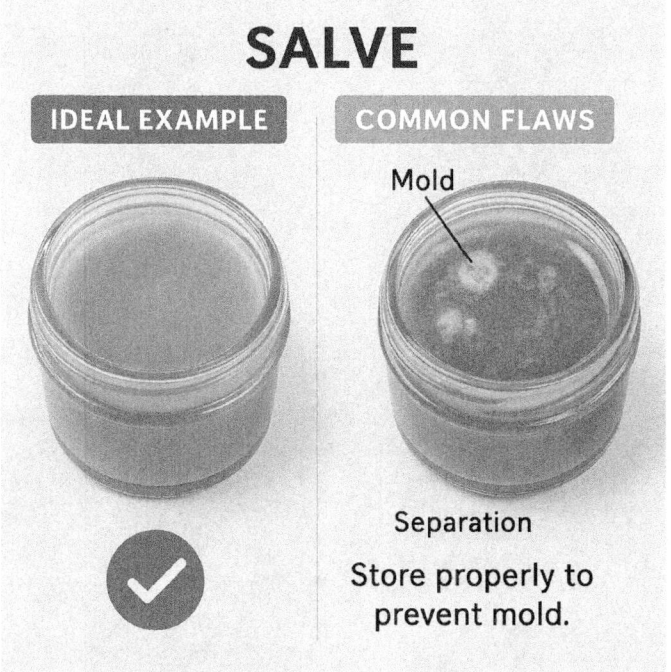

Herbal powders and capsules can be a bit trickier, especially when it comes to achieving the right grind. A good powder should be fine, dry, and evenly textured. Clumping or fibrous bits suggest an uneven grind or lingering moisture, which can affect potency and storage. We provide comparative images of ideal and flawed powders, including close-ups so you can compare texture directly.

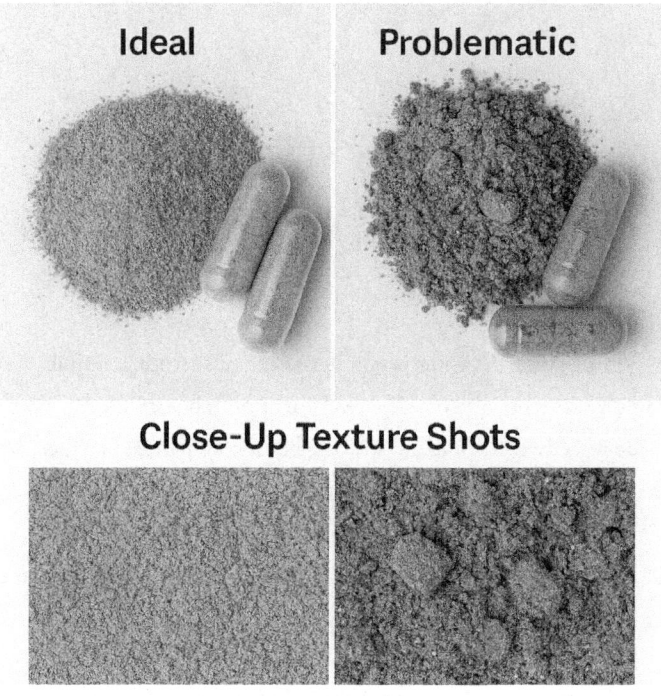

Homemade glycerites and treats bring another set of visuals. For example, it's not uncommon to see honey-based glycerites crystallizing over time—a natural occurrence that doesn't necessarily mean spoilage. Clear images illustrate normal vs. problematic honey separation. Treats like lozenges and herbal gummies are shown in a range of finishes: smooth and glossy, slightly cracked, or with minor surface bubbles—all acceptable and safe.

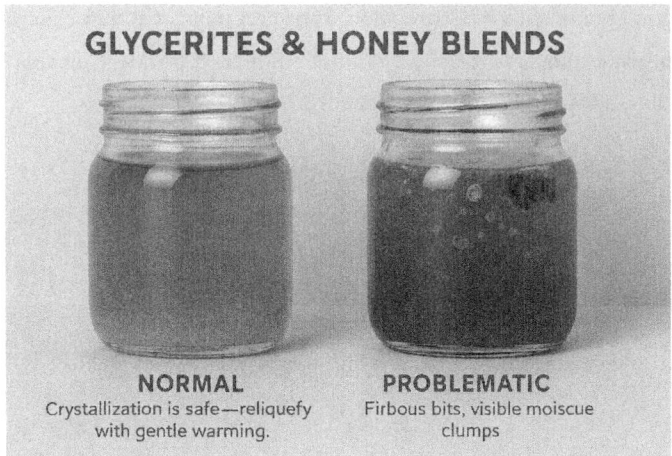

GLYCERITES & HONEY BLENDS

NORMAL
Crystallization is safe—reliquefy with gentle warming.

PROBLEMATIC
Firbous bits, visible moiscue clumps

Throughout the gallery, you'll also see numerous examples that demonstrate the "acceptable range" for appearance. Not every homemade remedy will come out looking like a commercial product, and that's okay. Color variation in tinctures due to different batches of herbs, or slightly uneven shapes in hand-formed herbal treats, are all signs of a genuine, handmade process. Embracing these natural variances builds both realism and pride into your DIY journey.

By familiarizing yourself with what successful DIY remedies look like across different types and stages, you develop a sharper eye for quality control. Whether it's distinguishing between acceptable quirks and signs of spoilage, or simply validating your process by comparison, these visuals help ensure your remedies are safe, potent, and made with confidence. In the next section, we'll walk through how to properly store each remedy to help maintain its visual and therapeutic integrity over time.

Safe Dosage and Administration—Personalized for Every Pup

From itchy skin to upset stomachs, many of the everyday ailments our dogs face can be gently and effectively managed with the right herbs. These natural remedies often work by addressing the root cause of discomfort—supporting the body's own healing processes—rather than simply masking symptoms. The beauty of herbal care is that it can be tailored to your dog's specific needs, offering relief that's both safe and sustainable.

In this chapter, we'll explore a carefully selected toolkit of herbs that every dog owner should know, along with the conditions they're most effective for. You'll learn which plants can soothe inflammation, ease digestion, boost immunity, promote healthy skin and coat, and more. We'll also cover practical tips for preparation and dosage, plus important safety notes to ensure each remedy benefits your dog without unwanted side effects.

By the end, you'll be equipped with a go-to reference of herbal allies for common canine health challenges—empowering you to respond quickly, confidently, and naturally when your dog needs support.

The "Doggy Dose" Calculator—Weight, Age, and Breed-Specific Guidance

When it comes to giving herbs and natural remedies to our four-legged companions, one size definitely does not fit all. Just as with conventional medicine, herbal dosing should be carefully calculated to suit each dog's unique characteristics. That's where the "Doggy Dose" Calculator comes in—a simple yet effective visual tool designed to guide you in determining the appropriate herbal dosage based on your dog's weight, age, and breed. Whether you're using chamomile for anxiety or turmeric for joint health, this calculator ensures that every drop, sprinkle, or spoonful is safe and effective.

Start by identifying your dog's weight category: toy (under 10 lbs), small (10–25 lbs), medium (26–50 lbs), large (51–90 lbs), or giant (over 90 lbs). These categories form the foundation of a customizable chart that adjusts dosage ranges proportionally to body mass. For instance, a toy breed might require only a few drops of an herbal tincture, while a giant breed could safely handle closer to a full teaspoon. Each weight bracket has been carefully scaled to reflect metabolic and physiological differences between breed sizes.

But weight isn't the only factor. Age plays a vital role in how a dog processes herbal supplements. Puppies, with still-developing organ systems, require more conservative doses, often one-quarter to one-half that of an adult dog in the same weight category. Senior dogs, especially those with liver or kidney sensitivity, may also need lower doses or slower escalation. Age-related digestive variability and slower metabolisms can impact how herbs are absorbed and utilized.

Breed type and known sensitivities further refine dosing. Brachycephalic dogs, like Bulldogs and Pugs, may have respiratory or metabolic sensitivities that warrant extra caution. Deep-chested or large-boned breeds, such as Great Danes and Greyhounds, metabolize substances differently and may need prolonged adjustment periods. Additionally, some breeds are genetically predisposed to liver issues (e.g., Scottish Terriers or Dobermans), which could affect herb selection and dosing frequency.

To bring the concept into clearer focus, let's look at a few real-world examples. Take a 12-pound senior Dachshund, for instance. If you wish to use chamomile tea to help with anxiety, you'd start with a quarter teaspoon of diluted tea mixed into food or administered via dropper, once or twice daily. As a senior, this pup may need slower titration, starting with just a few drops until tolerance is confirmed. On the other hand, a 70-pound adult Labrador suffering from arthritis can benefit from turmeric powder. In this case, a starting dose of 1/2 to 3/4 teaspoon of turmeric mixed with a carrier like coconut oil, once daily with food, would be appropriate. You can scale up incrementally while monitoring for gastrointestinal sensitivity or loose stools.

To make this practice easier, we've included both printable and digital versions of the Doggy Dose Calculator. The downloadable PDF includes blank fields for recording your dog's current weight, age, breed-specific notes, and dosage history. For those who prefer a high-tech option, a QR code in this book links to an interactive online calculator where you can input your dog's details for instant dosage recommendations tailored to common herbs.

By accounting for weight, age, and breed sensitivities, the "Doggy Dose" Calculator empowers you to confidently administer herbal remedies with precision and care. This thoughtful approach supports safety, increases effectiveness, and maintains the longstanding harmony between dogs and their natural medicine allies—paving the way for our next discussion: how to monitor your dog's response to herbal remedies over time.

Introducing New Herbs—The 3-Step Allergy and Sensitivity Protocol

When introducing any new herb to your dog's regimen, safety must always come first. Although herbs can offer wonderful support for overall health and wellbeing, dogs—like people—can react differently to substances based on their individual sensitivities. A thoughtful approach helps avoid unnecessary discomfort and, in rare cases, dangerous reactions. To ensure your dog tolerates a new herb well, follow this 3-Step Allergy and Sensitivity Protocol designed to ease them into the experience while giving you ample opportunity to observe and respond to their unique needs.

Start by offering a very small "test" dose—typically about one-quarter of the normal recommended amount based on your dog's size. It's best to mix this reduced dose into their food or a treat they enjoy. Then, wait and observe. The key is patience and close observation throughout the next 24 to 48 hours. During this period, be on the lookout for any reaction, no matter how small. If no adverse response is observed, you can move on to gradually increasing the dose. Over the next three days, raise the herb amount little by little until you reach the full recommended dose. If at any step your dog begins to show negative signs, stop administration and assess the symptoms before continuing.

So, what should you look for? Reactions can range from subtle to severe. Mild signs of an allergy or sensitivity may include increased scratching, licking of paws, watery eyes, or sneezing. These are often the body's first signals of irritation and should not be ignored. Moderate reactions may progress to vomiting, diarrhea, or visible hives—symptoms that warrant discontinuation of the herb and, depending on your dog's overall demeanor, may require a veterinarian consult. The most serious responses, while rare, include swelling of the face or muzzle, labored breathing, or even collapse—classic signs of anaphylaxis. These are critical emergencies that demand immediate veterinary attention.

To keep the process organized and support better decision-making, use a tracking method such as a "New Herb Trial Log." This simple, printable checklist allows you to record the name of the herb, date and dose given, observations after each dose, and any reactions encountered. It's also a helpful resource to bring to your vet if questions or concerns arise.

If your dog shows any sign of a reaction—whether mild or more serious—stop giving the herb immediately. For mild signs, monitoring at home may be sufficient, but if symptoms persist or escalate, call your veterinarian. In cases of more severe symptoms like swelling, breathing difficulties, or collapse, treat as a veterinary emergency. Most pet parents aren't equipped to handle anaphylaxis on their own, and a rapid response can be life-saving.

Introducing herbs properly is a valuable skill that ensures both safety and effectiveness. With this slow, deliberate approach—starting with a tiny dose, closely observing, and gradually increasing while documenting changes—you'll help your dog receive the support they need without unnecessary risk. In the next section, we'll explore how to build personalized herbal plans, taking into account your dog's condition, temperament, and lifestyle.

Mixing Methods—Making Remedies Palatable for Your Picky Eater

Even the most effective herbal remedies won't yield benefits if your dog refuses to take them. For pet parents with choosy companions, administering herbal treatments can feel like a daily battle. Fortunately, there are time-tested strategies for transforming herbal medicines from an unwelcome intrusion into a tasty treat, increasing the likelihood of consistent use and optimal results.

One of the most reliable techniques for masking bitter or unfamiliar herbal flavors is to blend them with strong-smelling, highly palatable foods. Dogs rely heavily on their sense of smell, so hiding herbs behind intense aromas can be surprisingly effective. Foods such as tuna, sardines, and bone broth are not only strong in scent but also rich in nutrients that complement herbal therapies. A spoonful of mashed sardines or a splash of warm, unsalted bone broth can disguise the taste of even the most pungent herbal powders or tinctures.

Another favorite among dog owners is xylitol-free peanut butter. This sticky, savory spread sticks to herbs well and can help deliver precise doses. Whether you're mixing powdered supplements, crushed herbal tablets, or drops of tincture, just a small amount of peanut butter can transform medicine time into a rewarding treat. Always double-check labels, as xylitol—a sugar substitute toxic to dogs—is found in some peanut butters.

Matching the right food supplement base to your specific herbal preparation can further increase success. Herbal teas, for example, are easily mixed into soft, absorbent bases like canned wet food or plain yogurt. This works particularly well with calming herbs like chamomile or nervines such as skullcap. Powders, on the other hand, blend nicely with thicker textures like canned pumpkin puree or mashed sweet potato, which not only mask flavor but also aid digestion. Here's a quick reference matrix of effective food pairings:

Herbal Form	Suggested Pairing
Herbal Tea	Wet food, plain yogurt, cottage cheese
Powder	Pumpkin puree, sweet potato, peanut butter
Tincture (alcohol-free)	Bone broth, sardines, mashed banana
Capsule (opened)	Tuna, egg, soft cheese, meat pâté

While experimentation is essential, it's equally important to avoid foods that are dangerous or problematic for dogs. Never use foods containing xylitol, chocolate, grapes, onions, garlic, or avocado, as these are toxic to dogs even in small amounts. Additionally, always monitor for food allergies or sensitivities—common allergens include dairy, certain meats, and grains. If your dog seems itchy, develops gastrointestinal upset, or loses interest in favorite foods after introducing a new carrier, it's wise to reassess and consult with a veterinarian.

Despite these methods, some dogs still resist herb-laden foods. In these cases, don't give up—adjust your delivery approach. Freezing herbal mixtures in silicone treat molds or ice cube trays can create cold, chewy treats that many dogs find irresistible. Hand-rolling herbal blends into mini balls using sticky bases like peanut butter and oats can also create portable, dose-controlled treats. Sensitive dogs may respond better to more neutral-tasting herbs, such as marshmallow root, oat straw, or alfalfa, which can be easier to introduce and gradually combined with stronger herbs as tolerance improves.

Creating herbal remedy routines your dog enjoys not only strengthens compliance but can become an enjoyable bonding moment. By experimenting with different carriers and techniques—and adjusting based on your dog's preferences—you'll transform medicine from a chore into a welcome part of your dog's daily life.

With the right mixing method and a little creativity, even picky eaters can benefit from the healing power of herbs. In the next section, we'll explore how to customize herbal formulas and dosing regimens based on your dog's individual needs and health goals.

Tracking Results—Journaling Templates and Symptom Logs

Consistent tracking is one of the most powerful tools when working with herbal remedies, especially when it comes to monitoring their safety, effectiveness, and any side effects that may arise. Without a reliable record-keeping system, it becomes incredibly difficult to assess how an herb is working, whether changes are due to the treatment or other external factors, or if adverse reactions are developing slowly over time. Thoughtful, regular journaling turns observations into actionable information.

Many symptoms, especially subtle ones or those that fluctuate—like digestive discomfort, mild lethargy, or changes in appetite—can easily go unnoticed in the busyness of daily life. Journaling creates a consistent checkpoint that helps you spot these less obvious shifts. It also prevents the human tendency to forget details or miss correlations, such as a delayed itchy rash that appears days after a new herbal blend is introduced. Journals serve as your objective memory, helping you detect patterns, progress, or problems that your brain alone might not retain accurately.

To make the process easy and manageable, this guide provides both printable and digital templates that you can use daily. The "Daily Herbal Log" is designed to track dosage, time of administration, the specific product used, and observable behaviors or physical responses. A separate "Symptom Change Chart" allows you to rate symptoms over time—whether you're dealing with skin conditions, joint stiffness, or gastrointestinal troubles—to see if there's gradual improvement or worsening. These tools transform your observations into data that can guide your next steps.

It's also important to record relevant variables outside of the remedies themselves. Diet changes, environmental stressors, or the introduction of new medications can all influence how herbs are metabolized or experienced by the body. For example, a log entry might read: "Added turkey to diet, started new herbal blend, stormy weather." While this may seem like an unrelated note at first, sudden behavioral or skin flare-ups may later correlate with protein sensitivity or barometric pressure drops, offering deeper insights.

Using these logs, you can troubleshoot inefficacies or emerging side effects by looking back through trends and pinpointing what changed when. If a remedy isn't working as expected, these records can help you adjust dosages, switch products, or decide when to discontinue use. They're also invaluable when sharing updates with your veterinarian or consultant—allowing for evidence-informed adjustments rather than guesswork.

When tracking physical conditions, such as dermatological issues, incorporating visual documentation is highly encouraged. Before-and-after photos taken in consistent lighting can reveal subtle progress that's hard to see day to day. For chronic issues like digestive upset or seasonal allergies, maintaining a timeline that illustrates flare-ups or resolution phases makes improvements tangible and easy to communicate.

In the journey with herbs, clarity comes from observation. By logging symptoms, dosing times, and environmental variables consistently, you build a reliable narrative of your experience—one that allows for safe, effective, and responsive herbal care.

Troubleshooting Dosage—What to Do if a Remedy Isn't Working

When using herbal remedies for dogs, it's not uncommon to encounter situations where a treatment doesn't seem to be producing the expected results—or worse, causes unwanted side effects. In these cases, understanding how to troubleshoot the remedy and dosage methodically can help avoid unnecessary risks while moving closer to an effective solution.

The first step is to double-check the dosage. Human error is common, and it's easy to misread labels, measure inaccurately, or confuse concentration strengths—especially with tinctures and extracts. Always refer to reliable dosage guidelines based on your dog's weight, and consider whether the current preparation (dried herb, tea, tincture, capsule) matches the recommended dosage form. Sometimes, concentrations vary between brands or products, increasing the chance of underdosing or overdosing.

Equally important is confirming correct herb identification. Even experienced pet owners may accidentally purchase the wrong species or variant, particularly when common names overlap. For example, "Chamomile" can refer to both German and Roman varieties, which have different chemical properties and effects. Always source herbal products from reputable suppliers and double-check botanical names to ensure accuracy.

If the dosage and identity are correct and your dog still isn't improving, it's helpful to consider the possibility that more time is needed. Some herbs work subtly and may require days or even weeks to show measurable effects. Tracking your dog's symptoms in a journal can provide insight into whether gradual progress is taking place, even if it's not immediately obvious.

Sometimes, the issue lies not with the herb itself but with the method of preparation. A dog who refuses to drink a tea may respond better to a tincture, powder mixed with food, or infusion added to bone broth. Flavor and absorption can significantly affect whether a remedy is effective. If your dog is refusing a particular dose form, switching to another method may make all the difference.

Adjusting the dosage is another step that requires careful consideration. If your dog experiences mild side effects—such as flatulence, loose stool, or increased thirst—it may be beneficial to reduce the dose temporarily. These symptoms can indicate that the body is adjusting or that the herb's potency may be a bit too strong for your dog's size or sensitivity. However, if you observe more severe effects like vomiting, lethargy, swelling, or difficulty breathing, discontinue the herb immediately and consult a veterinarian without delay.

In persistent cases where the remedy appears entirely ineffective or side effects are ongoing, it's time to seek professional help. A holistic or integrative veterinarian can evaluate whether the herbal supplement is interacting with other medications or if your dog has a condition that makes herbal use inappropriate. When you do visit the vet, come prepared: bring a log of all doses given (including dates, times, and observed reactions), photos of any visible symptoms, and a list of all supplements and medications your dog is taking. This documentation can help your vet pinpoint the issue more efficiently.

Keep a personal "do not retry" list for herbs your dog has reacted poorly to in the past. Sensitivities don't always show up immediately, and repeated exposure can lead to worsening symptoms. Cataloging these reactions protects not only your dog's current wellness but also serves as a vital point of reference for future care.

Ultimately, herbal remedies work best when used with thoughtful observation, accurate dosing, and a willingness to adapt. By approaching dosage troubleshooting systematically, dog owners can avoid common pitfalls and better support their dogs' health with safe, effective herb use.

Everyday Remedies for Common Canine Ailments

Every pet parent knows the heartache of seeing their beloved dog in discomfort — whether it's the incessant scratching from an allergy flare-up, the distress of an upset stomach, or the slow, stiff movement that comes with aging joints. While our first instinct may be to rush to the vet (and rightly so in serious cases), there are many mild to moderate conditions that can be gently treated with everyday, natural remedies—provided we know what to use and when.

In this chapter, we'll explore a holistic toolkit of safe, accessible, and effective remedies for common canine ailments. You'll learn how to relieve itching with pantry staples like oatmeal, how to use calming herbs for stress and anxiety, and which gentle supplements support joint health and digestion. We'll also discuss how to spot red flags that signal a trip to the vet is necessary—and when it's okay to treat at home.

If you've ever wished you had a trusted guide to handling those small but persistent health hiccups, you're in the right place. Let's tap into the power of nature, backed by sound veterinary principles, to help your dog feel better—every day.

Herbal Flea and Tick Prevention—DIY Sprays and Rinses

For dog owners seeking natural alternatives to chemical flea and tick preventatives, herbal remedies offer a promising solution rooted in tradition and supported by a growing body of anecdotal and scientific evidence. Carefully selected herbs like lemon balm, rosemary, and neem possess natural insect-repelling properties that make them ideal for canine use when thoughtfully prepared and safely applied. These botanicals not only deter pests effectively but also minimize the potential side effects associated with synthetic pesticides.

Lemon balm, known for its pleasant citrus scent and gentle astringent qualities, contains compounds that naturally repel insects. Rosemary, a Mediterranean herb rich in aromatic oils, has been shown to discourage fleas and ticks while imparting a refreshing scent. Neem oil, derived from the seeds of the neem tree, is perhaps the most potent of the three; it contains azadirachtin, a compound that interferes with the reproductive cycles of fleas and ticks, reducing their ability to thrive. However, while neem is powerful, it must be used with caution, particularly with pregnant or lactating dogs, as it may cause hormonal disturbances.

Creating your own flea and tick deterrents at home using these herbs can be both cost-effective and empowering. For a simple rinse, combine 1 cup of dried lemon balm with 2 cups of boiling water, allowing the herbs to steep for 30 minutes before straining. Add 1 tablespoon of apple cider vinegar, then allow the mixture to cool completely. Pour over your dog's coat after a bath, avoiding the eyes and mouth, to leave behind a subtle fragrance that naturally deters pests. Store any leftovers in the fridge and use within a week.

For a more potent spray designed for use on collars, bedding, or around the home, infuse 2 tablespoons of dried rosemary and 1 teaspoon of neem oil into 2 cups of boiling water. Once cooled and strained, pour the mixture into a spray bottle and shake well before each use. Because neem oil can be strong, it's important to dilute responsibly and avoid overuse. This spray should never be applied directly to the dog's skin unless directed by a veterinarian.

When using any natural remedy, safety is paramount. Always begin with a patch test—spray or rinse a small area of your dog's coat, wait 24 hours, and observe for signs of redness, excessive scratching, or irritation. Dogs with sensitive skin or known allergies may respond adversely even to natural ingredients, so caution and attentiveness are key. Regardless of the formulation, essential oils should never be used undiluted on canine skin, as they can cause chemical burns or systemic toxicity.

Pay attention to potential red-flag reactions. If you notice symptoms such as increased itching, red or inflamed skin, or unusual lethargy, discontinue use immediately and consult your veterinarian. As a general rule, topical herbal treatments should be reapplied once or twice a week during peak pest seasons, with adjustments based on your dog's exposure and skin sensitivity.

Natural flea and tick prevention through herbal sprays and rinses can be a safe and effective strategy when approached with knowledge and care. These DIY solutions offer an accessible way to incorporate preventive wellness into your dog's routine while fostering a chemical-free environment in your home. In the next section, we'll explore strategies for integrating herbal and conventional approaches to develop a comprehensive parasite control plan tailored to your dog's unique needs.

Soothing Itchy Skin and Hot Spots—Calendula, Oat, and Chamomile Protocols

Itchy skin and hot spots are common skin concerns many dog owners face, especially during allergy season or after exposure to irritants like pollen, dust, or insect bites. Fortunately, gentle herbal remedies like calendula, oat, and chamomile can bring soothing relief when applied correctly. These natural ingredients have anti-inflammatory, antimicrobial, and skin-calming properties that offer safe, effective support for mild irritations—right from the comfort of your home.

One of the most effective ways to use these herbs is through herbal rinses, compresses, and sprays designed to reduce redness, calm itchiness, and promote skin healing. For a general rinse that targets body-wide inflammation or widespread itching, an oatmeal and calendula tea blend can work wonders. Begin by combining 1 tablespoon of dried calendula flowers with 1/2 cup of finely ground colloidal oatmeal in a heatproof bowl. Pour 4 cups of boiling distilled water over the mixture, cover, and allow it to steep for 20 to 30 minutes. Once cooled to lukewarm temperature, strain the infusion through a fine mesh sieve or cheesecloth to remove plant material. The resulting liquid can be used as a gentle rinse after bath time or poured over affected areas and patted dry—no rinsing necessary afterwards.

To target localized itching—such as around the tail base, paw pads, or ears—a cool chamomile compress can be both calming and effective. Steep 2 tablespoons of dried chamomile flowers in 1 cup of boiling water for 15 minutes, then strain and cool. Soak a clean cloth or cotton pad in the cooled tea and apply it directly to the irritated area, holding it in place for 5–10 minutes. Repeat up to three times daily until symptoms subside. Chamomile's natural antihistamine and anti-inflammatory effects help reduce swelling and soothe histamine-induced itching.

Preparing these herbal treatments at home is simple and cost-effective. The key is to ensure proper steeping and straining to avoid leaving behind plant particles that could cause further irritation. Always use distilled or purified water to avoid introducing chlorine, chloramines, or other impurities. For sprays, pour the strained room-temperature herbal infusion into a clean spray bottle and store in the refrigerator for up to five days. Shake well before each use and discard if the mixture smells off or changes color.

While herbal care can be incredibly supportive for mild skin complaints, it's essential to recognize when professional veterinary intervention is needed. If a hot spot appears red, moist, and rapidly spreading, or is accompanied by pus, scabbing, or foul odor—signs of a bacterial infection—home remedies are no substitute for medical attention. Similarly, open wounds, extensive hair loss, or areas the dog persistently licks or bites at may require prescription treatments to prevent secondary complications. Monitor healing daily; gradual improvement with reduced redness, scabbing, and itching is a good sign. Any worsening warrants a vet visit.

Special attention should also be paid to dogs with known allergies or hypersensitive skin. While chamomile is soothing for many, dogs allergic to ragweed may experience reactions due to the plant family connection. In such cases, marshmallow root—an ultra-gentle demulcent herb—can be a suitable alternative. Steep 1 tablespoon dried marshmallow root in 1 cup of room-temperature distilled water for 4–6 hours for a cold infusion. Strain and use as a rinse or compress to hydrate and calm inflamed skin.

For chronic cases of sensitive skin, rotating between oat and calendula preparations can help prevent sensitization and maintain skin resilience over time. Always perform a small patch test when using a new herbal product, and observe your dog for any signs of worsening irritation or discomfort.

By incorporating these herbal protocols thoughtfully and knowing when to seek veterinary guidance, you can offer your dog natural, gentle relief from itchy skin and hot spots—supporting both comfort and long-term skin health in a safe, effective way.

Calming Anxiety—Herbal Chews, Teas, and "Rescue Remedy" Blends

For pet parents seeking natural methods to ease their dog's anxiety, herbal remedies have become a valuable complement to behavioral approaches and environmental management. Holistic veterinarians and herbalists often recommend specific calming herbs that show significant potential in reducing nervous tension in dogs. Among the most effective are valerian root, passionflower, and lemon balm—three botanicals with documented sedative and anti-anxiety properties safe for most dogs when used correctly.

Valerian (Valeriana officinalis) is one of the most well-known natural sedatives, often used to promote relaxation and reduce hyperactivity. It tends to be particularly helpful for dogs prone to excitement or insomnia-like restlessness. Passionflower (Passiflora incarnata) supports the nervous system by boosting levels of gamma-aminobutyric acid (GABA) in the brain, reducing brain activity associated with anxiety. Lemon balm (Melissa officinalis), a gentle and aromatic mint relative, shows both calming and digestive-soothing properties, making it a multi-benefit herb for anxious pups.

Incorporating these herbs into your dog's routine can be both simple and rewarding. One easy method is preparing homemade calming chews. A popular and palatable recipe combines 1 cup of oat flour, 1/2 cup of unsweetened peanut butter, 1 tablespoon of ground valerian root, and a splash of water to knead into a dough. Shape into bite-sized pieces and bake at 325°F for about 20 minutes. These chews can be stored in the refrigerator for up to a week or frozen for longer shelf life.

For a summer-friendly option, "calm cubes" made with lemon balm tea are soothing and refreshing. Brew a strong infusion using 1 tablespoon of dried lemon balm in 1 cup of hot water, steep for 10–15 minutes, then cool. Pour into silicone molds or ice cube trays and freeze. These are perfect before car rides or when you expect guests at home—situations that often trigger anxiety in dogs.

For acute stress scenarios such as thunderstorms, fireworks, or veterinary visits, a glycerite-based rescue remedy can be fast-acting and easy to administer. Combine equal parts glycerin and water, then add small amounts of valerian and passionflower extracts (consult dosage suggestions below). This blend can be given orally with a dropper about 20–30 minutes before the anticipated stressor. Always ensure the herbs used are alcohol-free and dosed appropriately.

Timing and dosing are crucial for herbal effectiveness and safety. For chronic or separation anxiety, daily low doses of calming herbs—administered in treats or teas—may have a cumulative effect, gently supporting the nervous system over time. In contrast, situational anxiety (like car trips or distant thunder) typically responds better to a moderate dose given 30–60 minutes prior to the event. As with any supplement, the key is observation: monitor your dog for signs of increased drowsiness, which might warrant lowering the dose. A small minority of dogs may show paradoxical excitement, particularly with valerian—restlessness, pacing, or hyperactivity—indicating that the herb may not be suitable in that case.

Safety always comes first when working with herbal preparations. While these herbs are generally well-tolerated, there are conditions under which caution is essential. Valerian, for instance, may interact with sedatives or anti-epileptic medications and should not be used in dogs who are pregnant, nursing, or have liver conditions. Passionflower and lemon balm are gentler but should still be introduced slowly. Red-flag symptoms to watch for include excessive sedation (difficulty waking), agitation, vomiting, or a dramatic change in behavior. If any of these appear, stop all herbal use and contact your veterinarian immediately.

In summary, soothing anxiety naturally with herbal chews, teas, and rescue blends offers a gentle way to support your dog's emotional health. With the right herbs, thoughtful dosing, and careful observation, you can create daily or situational solutions that align with holistic wellness while enhancing your dog's comfort during life's stressful moments.

Natural Joint Support—Turmeric, Boswellia, and Ginger for Arthritis

When addressing arthritis and joint discomfort in dogs, natural remedies are gaining recognition not only for their effectiveness but also for their gentle impact on the body compared to pharmaceuticals. Among the most researched and revered herbal allies in canine joint care are turmeric, Boswellia, and ginger. These botanicals offer significant anti-inflammatory and pain-relieving properties that can support long-term mobility and comfort in arthritic dogs.

Turmeric, particularly when prepared as "golden paste," is a powerful anti-inflammatory thanks to curcumin, its active compound. When combined with black pepper (which dramatically enhances its absorption) and a healthy fat such as coconut oil, turmeric becomes a highly bioavailable supplement for daily joint support. Many dog owners have seen marked improvement in stiffness and mobility after incorporating golden paste into their pets' routine over a few weeks.

Boswellia, also known as Indian frankincense, is another potent anti-inflammatory herb. It targets the same inflammatory pathways as some non-steroidal anti-inflammatory drugs (NSAIDs) without the harsh gastrointestinal side effects. When used alongside turmeric, Boswellia can provide enhanced relief, particularly in moderate to severe cases of arthritis. Ginger, with its warming and circulatory properties, supports joint health by reducing muscle tension and stiffness, especially helpful in colder seasons or in senior dogs.

A practical and enjoyable way to incorporate these herbs into a dog's diet is through homemade treats. One popular option is a turmeric and ginger-infused coconut oil treat. To make these, gently melt ½ cup of organic coconut oil, stir in 1 tablespoon of turmeric powder, ¼ teaspoon of ground ginger, and a pinch of freshly ground black pepper. Pour the mixture into silicone molds, allow it to cool, then store in the refrigerator for up to two weeks. Dose according to your dog's weight: start with ¼ teaspoon for every 10 pounds of body weight per day, and adjust as needed.

For owners who prefer a dry option, a powdered joint topper can be easily made by blending equal parts turmeric, ground ginger, and Boswellia powder. Sprinkle onto meals at the same dosage as the treats — introduce gradually and always monitor for tolerance.

Improvements from herbal joint support typically become noticeable after 2 to 4 weeks, with some dogs showing earlier results. Keeping a daily journal can help track signs of progress or regression. Note changes in your dog's range of motion, willingness to exercise, ability to rise after rest, and overall mood. During flare-ups or if new discomfort arises, temporarily increasing the frequency of dosing (within safe limits) may help, but always do so under veterinary guidance.

While these natural remedies can greatly enhance your dog's quality of life, they're not universally safe for all pets. Dogs with bleeding disorders or those taking blood-thinning medications should avoid turmeric due to its anticoagulant effects. Turmeric is also contraindicated in dogs with gallbladder disease, as it stimulates bile production. Animals already prescribed NSAIDs or corticosteroids should only use herbal supplements under veterinary supervision to avoid interactions or overdosing on anti-inflammatory effects.

Ultimately, if your dog continues to experience persistent limping, worsening pain, or shows signs of distress despite home care, it is crucial to consult your veterinarian promptly. Natural remedies should complement—not replace—a comprehensive healthcare plan.

Incorporating turmeric, Boswellia, and ginger into your dog's wellness regimen can offer noticeable relief from joint discomfort, improved mobility, and a higher quality of life. With safe preparation, consistent tracking, and informed care, these time-honored herbs can be powerful allies in managing arthritis the natural way.

Tummy Troubles—Gut-Soothing Teas for Gas, Diarrhea, and Nausea

Digestive upset is a common issue for pets and can leave both animals and caregivers feeling distressed. Whether it's bloating, gas, loose stools, or a bout of nausea, natural herbal teas can offer gentle and effective relief when used appropriately. Unlike pharmaceutical interventions, which can sometimes overcorrect or suppress natural gut functions, herbal teas nourish and soothe the digestive tract, often supporting recovery without harsh side effects.

Among the most trusted herbs for digestive wellness are slippery elm, marshmallow root, and ginger. Slippery elm, derived from the inner bark of the elm tree, forms a mucilaginous gel when brewed, which lines and coats the stomach and intestines. This protective layer can ease irritation while also reducing inflammation and supporting bowel regularity. Marshmallow root, similarly demulcent, helps calm inflamed mucous membranes and works particularly well in cases of mild diarrhea or stomach cramping. For nausea and gas, ginger is indispensable—its natural anti-inflammatory and carminative properties make it a go-to for queasy tummies, intestinal spasms, and sluggish digestion.

To make an effective gut-soothing tea blend, combine 1 teaspoon each of dried marshmallow root and slippery elm bark with ½ teaspoon of grated fresh ginger. Add the mixture to 2 cups of freshly boiled water and let steep for 15–20 minutes. Once cooled to room temperature, strain and serve in small amounts depending on your pet's size—start with a tablespoon for small pets and up to ¼ cup for larger ones. Unsweetened and unflavored, this formula can be administered directly via a spoon or mixed with food.

For a clever twist, try preparing marshmallow root and ginger "tummy cubes."" Start by steeping 1 tablespoon of marshmallow root and ½ tablespoon of grated fresh ginger in 1½ cups of hot water. After steeping, strain and pour the liquid into an ice cube tray. Once frozen, these cubes can be stored in a sealed container in the freezer and offered as needed. This method is especially handy when dealing with chronic issues or recurring travel-related nausea, as the cubes thaw quickly and can be mixed into a meal or slurped as a treat on a warm day.

While herbal teas are generally safe, especially when dosed conservatively, it's important to recognize when tummy troubles may be a sign of a more serious condition. Symptoms like persistent vomiting, listlessness, blood in the stool, black or tarry feces, or dehydration call for veterinary intervention, not an herbal remedy. If a symptom persists for more than 24 hours or worsens despite natural treatment, consult your vet without delay. Keep a "when to call the vet" checklist handy, including red flags like lethargy, uncontrollable diarrhea, or frequent vomiting, as early detection can often prevent more severe complications.

Integrating these healing herbs into your pet's diet can also work wonders for ongoing digestive support and prevention. For picky eaters, try mixing powdered slippery elm into a warm broth—bone broth or low-sodium chicken broth works well. The naturally thick texture blends beautifully and offers a gentle flavor enhancement. If your pet turns up their nose at ginger, try stirring a tiny pinch into canned pumpkin puree, which also offers fiber and soothing benefits for both constipation and diarrhea.

Supporting your pet's digestion with herbal teas can be both healing and preventative, offering a gentle line of defense against common ailments. By understanding how to prepare and serve safe, natural remedies—and knowing when medical help is necessary—you can respond confidently the next time a tummy issue arises.

Herbal First Aid for Minor Cuts, Scrapes, and Bug Bites

Minor wounds, scrapes, and bug bites are common occurrences for pets, especially active dogs who spend a lot of time exploring the outdoors. With the right herbal knowledge and a calm approach, many of these small injuries can be managed safely at home using gentle, natural remedies that support healing and reduce discomfort. Herbal first aid not only provides soothing comfort but also helps prevent infection and speeds recovery using plants known for their antimicrobial, anti-inflammatory, and skin-repairing properties.

For superficial scrapes and abrasions, a poultice made from calendula and plantain leaves can work wonders. Calendula, often referred to as "nature's skin healer," has soothing and antimicrobial properties, while plantain leaf, commonly found in backyards and parks, helps pull out toxins and encourages tissue regeneration. To create a basic poultice, crush or blend fresh calendula flowers and plantain leaves into a paste. Apply this directly to the affected area, cover with a piece of clean gauze, and secure it with medical tape or a loose-fitting bandage. Allow it to remain on the skin for 20–30 minutes, then rinse gently with lukewarm water.

In the case of bug bites or mild stings, a cool compress soaked in a witch hazel and chamomile infusion offers calming relief. Witch hazel acts as a natural astringent and anti-inflammatory agent, reducing swelling and irritation, while chamomile soothes itching and redness. To prepare the compress, steep chamomile flowers (or chamomile tea bags) in boiling water for 10 minutes. After the infusion cools to room temperature, add a splash of witch hazel. Soak a clean cloth in the mixture, wring out excess liquid, and hold it gently against the bite or irritated skin for several minutes. This can be repeated a few times a day as needed.

Proper wound care begins with gentle cleaning. Start with a homemade herbal rinse—such as a diluted calendula tea or a saline solution infused with lavender—to flush out debris and cleanse the area. After patting the wound dry with sterile gauze, apply a thin layer of herbal salve—made from ingredients like comfrey, calendula, and coconut oil—to encourage healing. Cover lightly with gauze and secure in place if needed. It's important to monitor the site daily, checking for any changes that could indicate infection.

Look out for warning signs that mean a veterinary visit is necessary. These include swelling that worsens rather than subsides, pus or foul-smelling discharge, noticeable pain when touched, signs of fever such as lethargy and warm ears, and wounds that don't begin to improve within a couple of days. Also, never attempt home treatment for puncture wounds, bites from other animals, or injuries near the eyes or mouth—these require prompt professional care.

To prevent your dog from licking or chewing on herbal treatments, which can reduce their effectiveness and sometimes introduce bacteria into the wound, simple barriers can help. Soft cones or inflatable collars allow your pet to move comfortably while stopping access to injuries. Dog booties can protect treated paws or legs, and wrapping the area with vet wrap can also help. Distraction is another useful tool—offering frozen treats, chew toys, or puzzles can keep your dog focused while the herbs do their work. Most topical remedies can be reapplied 2–3 times daily, especially after cleaning or if the dog has disturbed the dressing.

Using herbal remedies for minor wounds empowers pet owners to respond quickly and effectively with safe, plant-based solutions. With a watchful eye, proper technique, and a few clever tricks for keeping those remedies in place, you can support your dog's healing process naturally and confidently. Up next, we'll explore how to design a pet-safe herbal first aid kit, ensuring you're always prepared for life's little emergencies.

Enjoying the Journey with Your Dog So Far?

I hope you're finding this guide helpful as you explore safe, natural ways to care for your dog.

If the remedies, tips, and step-by-step instructions so far have sparked new confidence—or simply helped you see herbal care in a fresh light—I'd be truly grateful if you shared your thoughts in a quick review.

Your feedback not only helps other dog lovers discover the right resources, but it also encourages me to continue creating guides that are practical, trustworthy, and easy to follow.

It doesn't need to be long—just a few words about what you're finding most useful so far can make a real difference.

You can leave a review by clicking on this link or by scanning the QR code below:

Thank you for being part of this growing community of pet parents who want the very best for their dogs—naturally.

Now, let's keep going—there are so many more remedies and insights ahead.

Advanced Herbal Support for Chronic and "Left Out" Conditions

The real magic of canine herbalism often happens when individual herbs are combined into thoughtful, well-balanced formulas. By pairing plants with complementary actions, you can create remedies that address multiple aspects of a condition at once—supporting healing from different angles while minimizing potential side effects. But crafting these blends isn't just about mixing whatever you have on hand; it requires an understanding of each herb's strengths, limitations, and interactions.

In this chapter, we'll walk through the principles of formulating safe, effective herbal blends for dogs. You'll learn how to choose herbs that work synergistically, balance potent ingredients with gentler supporting herbs, and adjust proportions to fit your dog's size, age, and overall health. We'll cover the most common preparation methods—from tinctures and teas to salves and poultices—along with guidelines for proper storage and shelf life.

By the time you finish, you'll have the knowledge and confidence to create herbal formulas tailored to your dog's unique needs, ensuring that every blend you make is both safe and effective for long-term wellness.

Immune Support for Allergies and Autoimmune Conditions

The canine immune system serves as a complex and intelligent defense network, designed to protect the body from pathogens, allergens, and internal threats like cancerous cells. But when this system becomes unbalanced, it can respond improperly—either too aggressively, or by targeting the body's own tissues. In dogs, two of the most challenging manifestations of immune system misbehavior are allergies and autoimmune conditions. Though often confused, these issues stem from very different types of immune dysfunction and require nuanced, supportive care.

Allergies in dogs, including common seasonal or environmental allergies, represent a hypersensitivity reaction—essentially, the immune system overreacts to harmless substances like pollen or dust mites. Dogs may exhibit itching, red or watery eyes, ear infections, sneezing, or inflamed skin. In contrast, autoimmune conditions, such as autoimmune hemolytic anemia (AIHA) or lupus, occur when the immune system mistakenly identifies the body's own cells or organs as threats and attacks them. These disorders often present more systemically, with symptoms like sudden lethargy, fever, pale gums, or joint swelling.

Understanding the distinction is critical. Conventional treatments often rely on immunosuppressive drugs, which shut down portions of the immune system to reduce symptoms. While sometimes necessary, this approach can leave the dog vulnerable to infections and comes with long-term risks. An alternative, and often more sustainable approach, is immune modulation—encouraging the immune system to function more appropriately rather than simply suppressing its activity. This is especially important with chronic conditions, where prolonged suppression can take a toll on overall health.

Several botanicals have demonstrated gentle yet effective support for modulating the immune response in dogs. Among the most helpful is nettle leaf (Urtica dioica), known for its natural antihistamine properties. Rich in bioactive compounds, nettle works by stabilizing mast cells and reducing histamine release, which helps alleviate allergy symptoms like itching and redness—especially during high pollen seasons.

Reishi mushroom (Ganoderma lucidum) is another powerful ally. Revered in traditional Eastern medicine, reishi has adaptogenic, anti-inflammatory, and immune-regulating properties. It does not stimulate the immune system aggressively but rather helps bring it into balance, making it particularly useful for dogs with chronic allergic responses or mild autoimmune tendencies. Its polysaccharides and triterpenes work synergistically to calm inflammatory pathways while supporting normal cellular immunity.

Licorice root (Glycyrrhiza glabra) is often used as a short-term option during acute flares for its potent anti-inflammatory and soothing effects on mucous membranes and the skin. However, this herb must be used with caution. In dogs prone to heart or kidney disease, or those on medications that influence cortisol or potassium levels, licorice can increase water retention and blood pressure. It is best used under professional guidance for short durations only.

For pet parents looking to implement a holistic protocol, several strategies can be combined for both immediate relief and long-term immune support. A balanced rotating schedule of nettle and reishi, for example, can be cycled over 4–6 weeks to reduce the risk of tolerance and ensure continued efficacy. This approach allows time for the immune system to recalibrate without overwhelming the dog with constant herbal stimulation.

A simple antihistamine tea can also be prepared at home to help soothe symptoms of environmental allergies. Combine equal parts dried nettle, chamomile, and calendula flowers. Steep in hot water for 10–15 minutes, cool completely, and serve as a topper on food or in place of water (pending taste acceptance). This blend can calm itchy skin, reduce eye irritation, and support internal detoxification.

As beneficial as herbal therapies are, they must be used with careful observation and responsibility. Dogs with underlying conditions or on medications may experience herb-drug interactions. For instance, as mentioned, licorice should never be used in dogs with cardiac or renal issues without veterinary supervision. Additionally, pet parents should remain watchful for "red flag" symptoms that demand immediate veterinary intervention. These include swelling of the face or lips (which may indicate anaphylaxis), sudden collapse, pale gums, labored breathing, or extreme lethargy—particularly in dogs with suspected autoimmune disease.

Symptom	Potential Cause	Action Needed
Facial swelling	Allergic reaction/anaphylaxis	Immediate vet care
Sudden collapse	AIHA or anaphylaxis	Emergency vet visit
Pale gums	Blood cell destruction (AIHA)	Urgent evaluation required
Difficulty breathing	Severe allergy or lung issue	Emergency response needed
Persistent vomiting	Adverse herb reaction/flare-up	Contact veterinarian

By approaching immune-related conditions with a focus on modulation rather than suppression, and integrating carefully selected, evidence-backed herbs, dogs can enjoy greater relief and better resilience. With proper cycling, observation, and guidance, natural remedies can play a valuable role in supporting the canine immune system—gently guiding it back into balance and keeping our companions thriving.

Bladder and Urinary Tract Health—Cranberry, Marshmallow, and Beyond

Bladder and urinary tract issues are common in dogs, particularly as they age or experience other health stressors. The most frequently encountered concerns include recurrent urinary tract infections (UTIs), urinary crystals and stones (urolithiasis), and urinary incontinence. These conditions can cause significant discomfort and, if left unaddressed, may lead to more serious complications such as kidney infections or bladder damage.

Recognizing the signs early is key. Infections often present with symptoms such as frequent urination, accidents in the house, straining to urinate, licking at the urinary opening, or urine that appears cloudy or foul-smelling. Irritation or inflammation without actual bacterial infection—a condition sometimes referred to as sterile cystitis—may mimic symptoms of a UTI. In contrast, crystals or bladder stones can cause more severe discomfort, hematuria (blood in urine), or even urinary obstruction, especially in male dogs due to their narrower urethral anatomy. Understanding whether you're dealing with infection, inflammation, or obstruction is critical, as treatment strategies differ and mismanagement can delay recovery.

Among natural support options, cranberry and marshmallow root are two of the most talked-about herbs for maintaining urinary tract health, each with distinct modes of action. Cranberry's effectiveness lies in its ability to prevent bacteria, particularly E. coli, from adhering to the bladder walls through compounds called proanthocyanidins (PACs). While useful in prevention, cranberry is not a substitute for antibiotics during active infections. Furthermore, its acidifying effect on urine may not benefit all dogs—especially those prone to calcium oxalate stones, where excessive urine acidification can aggravate stone formation.

Marshmallow root, on the other hand, acts as a demulcent—coating and soothing the mucosal lining of the urinary tract. This makes it particularly helpful in cases of irritation or discomfort, whether from a mild infection, crystals, or post-treatment inflammation. Taken as a cold infusion, it delivers mucilage-rich, anti-inflammatory support without irritating sensitive systems.

A simple herbal tea blend combining these two can be a gentle daily preventive for dogs prone to UTIs:

> Cranberry-Marshmallow Root Tea (For Maintenance Support)
> - 1 teaspoon dried marshmallow root

- 2 tablespoons unsweetened dried cranberry pieces or concentrate (no added sugar or artificial sweeteners)

- 2 cups cool, filtered water

Let the marshmallow root steep in the cool water overnight (8–12 hours). Strain, then add the cranberry. Serve up to ¼ cup daily to a medium-sized dog, adjusting for size (e.g., 1–2 tablespoons for small dogs, up to ½ cup for large dogs).

When using marshmallow root powder as a supplement in food, dosages should be tailored by weight. Here's a general guideline for use as a demulcent:

Dog Weight	Marshmallow Root Powder Daily Dose
Under 20 lbs	⅛ teaspoon
20–50 lbs	¼ teaspoon
Over 50 lbs	½ teaspoon

Always mix into wet food or moistened kibble to allow for proper mucilage activation and absorption.

Helpful daily habits can make a tremendous difference for dogs predisposed to urinary issues. Keeping your dog well-hydrated dilutes the urine and flushes out irritants and bacteria before they have a chance to take hold. Encourage fluid intake with nutritious herbal broths—vegetable broth infused with parsley, celery, or corn silk can be appealing and mildly diuretic. You can also add water directly to meals or offer ice cubes soaked in mild herbal tea for enrichment and hydration.

For dogs with a history of delicate bladder linings or crystal formation, low-dose marshmallow root powder mixed into wet food can provide ongoing support. Look for high-moisture foods (e.g., fresh or canned diets) and avoid foods high in synthetic vitamin C, which may increase calcium oxalate risk in genetically predisposed breeds like Miniature Schnauzers, Yorkies, or Bichons Frises.

While these remedies are valuable tools for maintenance and mild support, it's vital to remain vigilant about safety. Not all herbs are appropriate when kidney function has been compromised—avoid herbs with diuretic or alkaloid-rich profiles (like uva ursi) in dogs with known kidney disease unless under veterinary guidance. More importantly, any signs of urinary obstruction or systemic illness demand immediate veterinary attention.

Watch for these red flags:

- Blood in the urine

- Frequent straining without producing urine

- Signs of pain or whimpering during urination

- Lethargy, vomiting, or loss of appetite alongside urinary changes

These symptoms could indicate anything from urethral blockage to kidney involvement and should never be managed at home.

Integrating herbs like cranberry and marshmallow root can play a valuable role in maintaining urinary comfort and reducing the recurrence of mild UTIs or inflammatory episodes, but they're not a substitute for medical care when needed. With thoughtful use and proactive daily strategies—hydration, gentle supplementation, and dietary mindfulness—dog guardians can help support long-term bladder health while being prepared to escalate appropriately when symptoms advance.

Up next, we'll explore herbal strategies for liver and detox support, focusing on how to safely assist your dog's natural cleansing pathways without overburdening such a vital organ.

Herbal Liver and Detox Support—Safe Cleansing for Sensitive Dogs

The liver is one of the most vital organs in a dog's body, tasked with filtering toxins, processing medications, and breaking down metabolic waste. In an increasingly chemical world where pets are exposed to environmental pollutants, processed foods, and long-term medications, providing liver support—especially for sensitive or chronically ill dogs—has become not just beneficial, but essential. However, it's crucial to distinguish between supporting the liver gently and engaging in aggressive detox protocols, which can sometimes do more harm than good.

In human wellness trends, the term "detox" is often associated with quick, dramatic cleanses. Transplanted onto our pets, this approach can lead to unintended consequences. Dogs have much smaller systems, and unlike humans, they can't communicate subtle discomfort. Over-cleansing or utilizing potent herbal blends without understanding their effects may burden the liver instead of helping it. Some commercial detox products designed for pets are overly aggressive or improperly dosed, potentially triggering diarrhea, lethargy, or vomiting—clear signs that the body is being pushed too hard. For dogs, particularly those with health sensitivities or chronic conditions, gentle, supportive liver care should always take precedence over any rapid detox attempt.

Several well-researched herbs offer dog-safe liver support when used appropriately. Chief among them is milk thistle, specifically its active compound silymarin. This antioxidant-rich flavonoid helps protect liver cells from toxin-induced damage and promotes regeneration. Milk thistle is particularly beneficial for dogs taking long-term medications like NSAIDs, anti-seizure drugs, or steroids. For dosing, a general rule is 50–100 mg of silymarin per 10 pounds of body weight, commonly administered once or twice daily depending on the severity of liver stress and veterinary advice. Always ensure the product used is formulated specifically for pets or confirmed safe with a vet before use.

Dandelion root, another gentle detoxifier, works by stimulating bile production and aiding healthy digestion, especially in dogs with signs of sluggish or fatty digestion, such as gassiness or dull stools. A mild dandelion root tea—steeped, cooled, and given with meals—can help tone the liver without overstimulation. Artichoke leaf extract is a lesser-known but powerful aid, working synergistically with milk thistle to enhance bile flow and support lipid metabolism.

To ensure safety and effectiveness, liver support should be introduced through structured, phased protocols. A helpful approach for dogs on chronic medication is a four-week liver support plan. Begin with gradually adding herbal support such as milk thistle and dandelion root during week one. Monitor for changes in energy, appetite, or stool quality. If well-tolerated, continue the regimen for three more weeks, then pause for a week to reassess. Liver support herbs are best used in cycles—supporting the organ in phases rather than continuously—to avoid overuse and allow the liver to function naturally between cycles.

While liver support is generally low-risk when approached thoughtfully, there are critical exceptions. Dogs exhibiting symptoms such as yellowing of the eyes or gums, persistent vomiting, bloated abdomen, or dark urine must see a veterinarian immediately. These signs may indicate serious liver or gallbladder conditions such as bile duct obstruction, hepatitis, or liver failure—not cases for home detox strategies. Additionally, any dog with a history of pancreatitis or current digestive instability should not be placed on herbal support without veterinary guidance.

To help navigate this delicate balance, the following chart clarifies when liver support at home might be safe versus when professional help is vital:

Symptom or Condition	Safe for Home Support?
Dog on long-term medication, stable	✓ Yes (with monitoring)
Occasional sluggish digestion	✓ Yes (e.g., dandelion tea)
Yellowing of eyes or gums	✗ No – See vet immediately
Active vomiting, diarrhea, or lethargy	✗ No – Requires evaluation
Known liver disease with recent lab work	✓ Yes (alongside vet care)
Appetite loss more than 48 hours	✗ No – Possible emergency

Gentle liver and detox support, when applied knowledgeably and responsibly, can help dogs better process environmental toxins, medications, and metabolic waste. The key is always to proceed carefully, observe closely, and never mistake herbal remedies for solutions to urgent medical issues. With the right approach, sensitive dogs can benefit greatly from thoughtful, periodic liver support as part of a holistic health regimen.

Heart Health—Hawthorn and Motherwort for Senior Dogs

As dogs reach their senior years, it's not uncommon for their hearts to experience wear and tear just like in aging humans. Chronic cardiac conditions, particularly degenerative valvular disease and the early stages of congestive heart failure, become increasingly prevalent in geriatric dogs. These conditions can progress slowly, often causing symptoms such as persistent coughing (especially at night or after exercise), reluctance to engage in physical activity, and even occasional fainting spells due to poor circulation. While veterinary guidance and medication are crucial in managing these conditions, herbal allies like hawthorn and motherwort can offer gentle, supplemental support when used responsibly.

Hawthorn (Crataegus spp.) is widely recognized in herbal medicine for its affinity with the cardiovascular system. Its berries, leaves, and flowers contain powerful antioxidants, flavonoids, and bioactive compounds that support both the integrity of blood vessels and overall cardiac function. In human and veterinary herbalism, hawthorn is often used to enhance circulation, stabilize blood pressure, and mildly strengthen the heart's pumping action. For senior dogs, a daily syrup made from hawthorn berries can be a comforting and effective way to administer this supportive remedy. To make the syrup, simmer 1 cup of dried hawthorn berries in 2 cups of water for 45–60 minutes, strain, then mix with 1 cup of vegetable glycerin or honey. Administer 1 tsp per 25 lbs of body weight daily, mixed with food.

Motherwort (Leonurus cardiaca), meanwhile, plays a different but complementary role. Traditionally used to calm heart palpitations and gently lower blood pressure, motherwort is a low-dose herb that can support dogs experiencing increased cardiac workload or mild anxiety around breathing discomfort. It is most effective in tincture form, with a conservative dose of just 1–3 drops per 20 lbs of body weight, 1–2 times daily. Due to its potential to lower blood pressure, caution is warranted in dogs who already have low readings, and its use should always be discussed with your veterinarian—especially if your dog is on cardiac medications.

When integrating herbs like hawthorn and motherwort into a treatment protocol that includes veterinary prescriptions, coordination with your veterinarian is essential. These herbs exert physiological effects that could interact with medications such as beta blockers or digitalis derivatives. Use the following general protocol with vet approval: begin with the lowest effective herbal dose, space the herbal and pharmaceutical doses several hours apart, and monitor the dog's response carefully over a two-week period before adjusting.

> Important Note - Do not use hawthorn or motherwort if your dog is on digitalis (e.g., Digoxin) or beta blockers without veterinary supervision.

Regular monitoring is essential any time you add a new component to your dog's cardiac care plan. Watch for any signs of gastrointestinal discomfort (such as vomiting or diarrhea), a notable slowing of the heartbeat (bradycardia), or signs of general malaise after starting herbs. Adjustments to the dosing—or discontinuation—may be necessary depending on your dog's individual tolerance and concurrent therapies.

There are also limits to what herbal support can do. Herbs are not a substitute for emergency or critical care. Absolute contraindications for home herbal care include symptoms such as sudden collapse, severely labored breathing, marked decrease in exercise tolerance, or rapid unexplained weight gain—especially with signs of abdominal swelling, which may indicate fluid retention. In these cases, veterinary intervention is urgent.

A practical way to track your dog's cardiac status at home is by recording resting respiratory rate (RRR). When your dog is completely asleep, count the number of breaths per minute. A number above 30 consistently, or a sharp increase from their typical baseline, may indicate worsening heart function—whether or not symptoms appear outwardly.

Hawthorn and motherwort offer gentle, time-honored support to senior dogs facing the natural slow-down of cardiac aging. When paired responsibly with veterinary care and monitored properly, they can improve quality of life and maintain comfort for beloved dogs in their golden years. As we shift into addressing more specific strategies for managing respiratory distress and fluid retention, the next section will expand on complementary herbs that play a role in easing the burden on an aging heart.

Herbal Approaches to Cancer Support—What's Safe, What's Not

When a beloved dog is diagnosed with cancer, many pet parents turn to complementary options in search of hope, relief, or just the feeling of doing everything possible. Herbal support can play a valuable role in a comprehensive cancer care plan, but it's important to understand that herbs are not a replacement for veterinary oncology. Instead, they can serve as a gentle, natural complement that may help improve quality of life, support the immune system, and ease side effects when carefully chosen and responsibly used. As always, honesty and compassion are key when managing expectations—herbal remedies are not cures, but they may offer comfort and resilience as your dog navigates treatment.

Among the most well-studied and widely used herbal ingredients in canine cancer support are medicinal mushrooms such as shiitake, maitake, and reishi. These fungi are rich in beta-glucans and other compounds that modulate immune activity, potentially enhancing the body's natural defenses without overstimulating them. Medicinal mushroom powders can often be safely integrated into meals, and many dogs tolerate them well. Pet caregivers have reported improvements in energy, appetite, and overall vitality during treatment courses when these mushrooms are included.

Turmeric, specifically its active component curcumin, is another herbal option with documented anti-inflammatory properties. Chronic inflammation has been linked to cancer progression, and curcumin may help mitigate this process when used appropriately. While canine bioavailability of curcumin is limited, combining turmeric with a healthy fat source and a pinch of black pepper can improve absorption. Golden paste recipes, commonly used in integrative pet practices, provide a palatable way to administer turmeric.

Another herb sometimes used in cancer support is astragalus, a traditional Chinese remedy known for immune-boosting properties. However, caution is warranted: astragalus should not be used in dogs with autoimmune disease or active fevers, as it may further stimulate inappropriate immune responses. Always consult a veterinary professional familiar with herbal medicine before introducing this or any herb, especially in medically complex cases.

Integrating herbal therapies alongside conventional treatments like chemotherapy, radiation, or pain medications requires thoughtful coordination. Some herbs can interfere with drug metabolism or potentiate side effects, so open communication with your veterinarian is essential. For example, St. John's wort, although popular in human herbal medicine, can alter drug metabolism in the liver and should be avoided. Likewise, comfrey—due to its liver toxicity—and bloodroot, which can cause severe tissue damage and worsen wounds, are strictly off-limits, particularly in a cancer context.

If you're considering incorporating herbs at mealtime, start simple. A sample plan might include a scoop of reishi mushroom powder mixed into a warm, bland meal like boiled chicken and rice. Monitor your dog closely for signs of digestive upset and keep detailed notes. Creating a documentation template to record daily observations—appetite, stool quality, energy levels, and any treatment side effects—can provide valuable insights and assist your veterinarian in adjusting the care plan.

Perhaps most importantly, stay alert to red flags. Any signs of rapid tumor growth, internal or external bleeding, sudden weight loss, or dramatic behavior changes are cause for immediate veterinary attention. Herbal interventions under such circumstances may delay critical care or inadvertently complicate treatment. A simple flowchart—starting with, "Has your dog had a veterinary cancer diagnosis?" and progressing through checkpoints like "Is your dog on medication?" or "Has there been a change in symptoms?"—can help guide decision-making and underscore when professional input is non-negotiable.

In summary, herbal approaches can offer meaningful support for dogs with cancer, especially when used judiciously, transparently, and as part of an integrated care plan. When partnered with conventional medicine and guided by a qualified veterinary professional, the right herbs may ease discomfort and strengthen your dog's overall resilience during one of life's hardest battles.

Easing Cognitive Decline—Herbs for the Aging Canine Brain

As dogs enter their senior years, it's not uncommon for them to experience a gradual decline in cognitive function—a condition widely recognized as canine cognitive dysfunction (CCD), or more informally, "doggie dementia." Much like Alzheimer's in humans, CCD is a neurodegenerative condition that affects memory, learning, and behavior. Pet owners may begin to notice subtle changes: a previously house-trained dog may start having indoor accidents, or a once-confident companion may seem disoriented, getting stuck behind furniture or struggling to recognize familiar surroundings. Nighttime anxiety, vocalizing, and restlessness are also common, disrupting both the dog's sleep patterns and their human family's routines. These shifts can be deeply distressing, not just for the caregiver but also for the dog whose world suddenly seems less predictable and secure.

Supporting brain health in senior dogs involves a multi-faceted approach—routines, enrichment, veterinary care, and importantly, natural aids that may help maintain cognitive function. Several herbs with traditional and scientifically studied neuroprotective properties have gained attention for their potential to ease symptoms of CCD and support quality of life during the aging process.

Ginkgo biloba is one such herb, often heralded for its ability to improve cerebral circulation and protect neurons from oxidative damage. In dogs, ginkgo is typically administered in tincture form, with dosage carefully adjusted according to the dog's weight—usually around 1 drop per 10 pounds, twice daily. While promising, it's critical to avoid ginkgo in dogs with bleeding disorders or those on anticoagulant medications, as it may increase the risk of hemorrhage.

Gotu kola, another revered herb in traditional medicine systems, has long been regarded as a "brain tonic." Its compounds are thought to promote mental clarity and reduce anxiety, which can be particularly helpful for older dogs exhibiting increased nervousness or confusion. Available as a powdered herb or capsule, gotu kola can be mixed directly into food or incorporated into homemade treats.

For dogs that become anxious or agitated in the evening hours—a common CCD hallmark—lemon balm provides gentle calming effects. Its mild sedative properties can support sleep and reduce nighttime restlessness. Brewed as a weak tea and added to the water bowl at bedtime, lemon balm can help create a more peaceful transition to sleep without the grogginess of pharmaceutical sedatives.

In practice, integrating these herbs into a senior dog's routine can be both simple and enjoyable. A weekly "brain treat" might include a blend of powdered ginkgo and gotu kola mixed with oat flour, peanut butter, and a touch of honey, rolled into small bites and refrigerated. This approach not only delivers the herbs in a tasty format but also provides a food-based ritual the dog can look forward to.

Lemon balm tea, brewed weak (one teaspoon dried lemon balm per cup of hot water, steeped and cooled), can be added to a dog's water bowl in the evening—about a quarter cup depending on size. Always ensure fresh water is available separately, especially when introducing herbal additives for the first time.

While these herbs can offer gentle and effective support, it's essential to monitor progress and remain alert to changes. Keep a daily log of sleep duration and quality, episodes of disorientation, appetite variation, and engagement in familiar tasks or environments. Over time, this kind of tracking will help determine whether an herbal protocol is improving your dog's life or if adjustments are needed. In general, mild benefits may appear within two weeks, with more observable improvement often evident after 4 to 6 weeks of consistent use.

Ultimately, the goal in herbal support for canine cognition is not reversal but stabilization—to help senior dogs feel more at ease, maintain connection with their world, and enjoy their golden years with comfort and dignity. As we explore the broader toolkit of natural care for aging dogs, understanding how herbs can gently support brain function lays the groundwork for a more holistic approach to senior pet wellness.

Integration with Modern Pet Lifestyles

Knowing which herbs to use is only half the equation—how you give them to your dog can make all the difference in whether the remedy works as intended. Dogs vary widely in size, taste preferences, and tolerance, so the method and dosage need to be tailored to each individual. Too little, and you may not see results; too much, and you risk side effects. The goal is to deliver the right amount, in the right way, so your dog gets the full benefit without unnecessary stress or resistance.

In this chapter, we'll explore the different ways to administer herbal remedies, from adding tinctures to food, to brewing herbal teas, to applying topical preparations for skin issues. You'll learn how to measure dosages based on your dog's weight, when to give herbs with food versus on an empty stomach, and tips for getting even the pickiest dogs to take their medicine. We'll also cover how to watch for changes—both positive and negative—so you can adjust quickly if needed.

By the end, you'll feel confident in not only choosing the right remedy but also delivering it in a way that's safe, stress-free, and effective for your dog.

Batch-Prep and Time-Saving Herbal Routines for Busy Households

In busy households, time often feels like the most limited resource—especially when caring for both humans and pets. Fortunately, herbal care does not need to be a labor-intensive, daily endeavor. With just a bit of planning, herbal remedies can be prepared in larger batches, stored properly, and integrated into daily routines effortlessly. Batching saves time, ensures consistency, and reduces stress for caregivers juggling multiple responsibilities.

To begin, making weekly or bi-weekly batches of common remedies like teas, tinctures, and salves can significantly reduce the time spent preparing treatments each day. For instance, a calming herbal tea blend made from chamomile, lemon balm, and oat straw can be steeped in a mason jar and stored in the refrigerator for up to four days. Simply pour into your dog's food or water dish as needed. Tinctures can be pre-mixed into a weekly dropper bottle in advance based on your dog's daily dosage. For topical care, making salves—like a calendula and comfrey ointment—once a month and storing them in small silicone jars makes it easy to grab and apply as part of your bedtime pet care routine.

Proper storage is essential to maintain the potency and safety of herbal remedies. Using high-quality glass jars with airtight lids protects dried herbs and teas from contamination and moisture. Silicone freezer trays work beautifully for freezing single doses of herbal broths or decoctions—pop one out the night before and it's ready to use by morning. Labeling is key: clearly mark each container with the herb blend name, expiration date, and intended purpose. Color-coded stickers can help distinguish between internal and external-use remedies at a glance. Consider designating one small shelf or portable basket as your family's "herbal care station," keeping everything organized and within easy reach.

For families constantly on the go, a consistent herbal care schedule is just as important as the remedies themselves. A printable "weekly herbal planner" can help track your dog's herbal intake and application schedule within your family's existing routines. For example, chamomile drops for calming can align with bedtime, while turmeric paste for inflammation might be added to the morning meal. Checklists broken down by morning, afternoon, and night keep things simple. Planners can be posted on the fridge, printed as part of your pet health binder, or stored digitally on your device for quick reference.

Real-world herbal care often requires clever time-saving strategies, especially in multi-pet homes or families with unpredictable work schedules. One method is crafting multi-use herbal bases—like a turmeric-coconut oil blend that can be used both as a food additive for inflammation and as a topical balm for sore joints. Another helpful strategy is using smartphone apps to set medication reminders and dosage alerts—ensuring no dose is missed, even during hectic school runs or unexpected late nights. Some pet owners use labeled pill organizers to pre-measure dry herb capsules or pressed powder doses for the entire week, requiring only a quick grab-and-go at each meal.

Whether you're managing remedies for an elderly dog with arthritis, juggling school runs and pet care, or simply seeking to streamline your weeknights, these batching and scheduling techniques put herbalism on autopilot—without compromising on care and quality. Through thoughtful preparation and a few strategic tools, you can ensure that your dog consistently receives the gentle support of herbs in a way that fits seamlessly within your family's lifestyle. This practical rhythm not only nurtures your dog's health but fosters peace of mind for everyone involved, paving the way for the next layer of safe and confident canine herbalism.

Travel Kits—On-the-Go Remedies for Road Trips and Boarding

Traveling with your dog, whether it's a long car ride or a temporary boarding stay, often involves new routines, unfamiliar environments, and potential stressors—for both you and your pup. Assembling a well-stocked, TSA-friendly herbal travel kit ensures your dog's health and comfort are supported on the go, whether you're headed to a lakeside cabin or dropping your furry friend off at a boarding facility. Tailoring the kit to your dog's specific needs and destination type allows you to pack confidently and manage common travel-related concerns with ease.

At the core of any herbal travel kit are three essential remedy categories: calming support, digestive aid, and first aid. For calming, consider including a small tincture bottle of chamomile, valerian, or passionflower to help soothe travel anxiety or separation stress during boarding. These can ease restlessness during long rides or kennel stays. For digestion, bring powdered slippery elm bark to address sudden bouts of diarrhea or upset stomach—common during travel transitions. A few ginger chews are helpful for motion sickness or nausea. For first aid, pack salves infused with calendula and comfrey to treat cuts, scrapes, or irritation from outdoor adventures. A few plantain leaf tea bags can double as topical compresses for insect bites or minor inflammation.

To keep your remedies safe, compact, and travel-appropriate, go for smart, portable packaging. Silicone squeeze bottles are ideal for liquids like tinctures or herbal washes, as they're flexible, leak-resistant, and pass TSA regulations for carry-ons. Mini tins are perfect for salves—lightweight, durable, and easy to label. For powdered herbs and teas, use sealable waterproof bags or reusable glass vials with screw lids, keeping labels intact to avoid confusion. If temperature extremes are expected, wrap sensitive items in reusable thermal pouches or store them inside insulated lunch bags to maintain potency.

If your dog will be cared for by someone else while you're away—such as a pet sitter, friend, or boarding staff—it's essential to communicate clearly about their herbal routine. Prepare a printed "herbal instruction card" detailing each remedy, when and how it should be given, and why it's used. Include any preferences your dog has, such as taking tinctures with their food or needing a pill pocket for powdered herbs. Discuss the herbal plan during the intake process, requesting that staff note it in your dog's file. Providing familiarity in their routine, even in your absence, helps ease both your dog's transition and the caregivers' responsibilities.

Travel sometimes involves unpredictable hiccups, so it's wise to be prepared for common remedy-related issues. For instance, store powdered herbs in double-sealed bags to prevent moisture damage in humid climates or meltwater exposure during winter trips. If your luggage is delayed or lost, keep a backup supply of your most essential remedies in your carry-on. In the unfortunate event a tincture spills en route, rinse the container thoroughly and wipe other kit items with herbal-safe wipes, then find a local natural market or pet store at your destination to replace what's lost whenever possible. For missed doses, simply resume the herbal plan at the next appropriate time without doubling up.

A well-prepared travel kit can turn unpredictable journeys into smoother, safer experiences for your dog and peace of mind for you. Whether it's a weekend drive or a longer boarding stay, having the right natural remedies accessible and well-communicated supports your dog's well-being—wherever the road may lead.

Mealtime Add-Ins—Blending Herbs with Food for Daily Wellness

Enhancing your dog's meals with medicinal herbs isn't just a comfort to their palate—it can also be a proactive step toward long-term health, greater vitality, and the prevention of chronic illness. Incorporating herbs into daily meals, in small, safe, and flavorful amounts, turns everyday feeding into an opportunity for wellness. Often referred to as "kitchen herbs," many of these plant-based additions are already hiding in your spice rack or produce drawer, ready to be put to good use. Parsley, for instance, offers more than a garnish—it's rich in chlorophyll, freshens breath naturally, and supports kidney health. Likewise, turmeric, known for its vibrant color and earthy flavor, plays a powerful anti-inflammatory role and supports joint health.

Integrating herbs into your pet's diet doesn't have to be complex. With awareness of appropriate dosages and palatable pairings, this can be as simple as sprinkling, mixing, or blending herbs into your dog's preferred meal style—be it kibble, raw, or home-cooked. To help guide consistent and safe use, the following list includes common herbs, their general benefits, dosage suggestions for medium-sized dogs (typically 30–50 lbs), and compatible food pairings:

Herb	Benefits	Suggested Daily Amount	Recommended Pairings
Parsley	Breath freshener, diuretic	½ to 1 tsp chopped, fresh	Mix into cooked or raw meals; sprinkle on wet kibble
Turmeric	Anti-inflammatory, antioxidant	¼ tsp powder with fat base	Blend with yogurt, bone broth, or golden paste
Nettle (dried)	Allergy support, joint health	½ tsp powder or crushed	Sprinkle over wet food or mix into ground meat
Ginger	Digestive aid, anti-nausea	⅛ to ¼ tsp powder	Combine with pumpkin puree or cook into bland diet meals
Rosemary	Antioxidant, circulatory support	Pinch dried or fresh	Add to stewed homemade meals or meat-based broths

Just as important as the health benefits is ensuring these additions are both enjoyable and digestible. Simple yet creative recipes can make herbs more appealing and increase compliance, especially for picky eaters. A popular go-to is dog-friendly broth cubes: simmer a blend of pet-safe bones and vegetables, then add herbs like parsley or turmeric before pouring into ice cube trays to freeze. These can be thawed at mealtime or served as cooling treats in warmer months. Herbal powders can also be blended into fermented bases such as goat milk or unsweetened yogurt, which not only enhance flavor and texture but also promote gut health. For an extra boost, consider stirring in probiotics or digestive enzymes to support nutrient absorption alongside the herbs.

For dogs that are skeptical when new flavors are introduced, transitioning gradually is key. Begin with a pinch of the chosen herb mixed into a favorite meal, and slowly work up to the full dose over several days. Using warm herbal broths as "gravy" over kibble can disguise the herb's taste while improving palatability. For pups with food sensitivities or allergies, substitute base ingredients accordingly—coconut or oat-based yogurts can stand in for dairy, and bone broth alternatives like mushroom broth can support dogs on special diets.

By strategically blending herbs into your dog's meals, you support health from the inside out—encouraging resilience, aiding digestion, reducing inflammation, and much more. With a thoughtful, flavorful approach, herbal nourishment becomes part of the daily routine—no fuss, just wellness at every bite. This sets the stage for deeper exploration into therapeutic herbal preparations and more targeted wellness strategies ahead.

Herbal Hygiene—Ear Washes, Tooth Powders, and Clean Paws

Maintaining your dog's hygiene is essential not only for their comfort but for their long-term health. Herbal hygiene offers a natural and gentle approach to regular grooming, using plant-based ingredients that support wellness while minimizing exposure to harsh chemicals and synthetic fragrances. Just like humans, dogs benefit from consistent oral care, clean ears, and healthy paws—herbal solutions make these routines soothing and safe.

Incorporating herbs into your dog's hygiene care provides preventative maintenance by reducing the risk of infections, irritation, and buildup. A simple herbal ear wash can help keep ears clean and itch-free, while an herbal tooth powder combats plaque without chemical additives. Likewise, paw soaks infused with natural astringents and moisturizers can both sanitize and heal the pads of your dog's feet, especially after long walks or exposure to rough terrain.

Creating your own herbal hygiene products at home is easier than it might seem. A chamomile and calendula ear rinse combines two gentle anti-inflammatory herbs that soothe and cleanse without stinging. To make it, steep one tablespoon each of dried chamomile and calendula flowers in a cup of hot distilled water. Let the mixture cool completely, strain it, and store in a clean dropper bottle for up to a week in the fridge. Use a cotton ball to gently apply the rinse to the outer ear canal—never pour liquid directly into the ear. This rinse is calming and helps prevent wax buildup and odors.

For oral care, a parsley and baking soda tooth powder offers a refreshing and effective solution. Finely chop 2 tablespoons of fresh parsley (a natural breath freshener and mild antimicrobial), and mix well with 1/4 cup of baking soda. Store the mixture in an airtight container, and use a fingertip brush or a small piece of gauze wrapped around your finger to apply. Gently rub the powder in small circles across the teeth and along the gum line. Aim for brushing a few times a week, depending on your dog's tolerance.

Cleaning your dog's paws not only removes dirt and allergens but also helps soothe cracked or irritated pads. A witch hazel and aloe soak is ideal, blending the cooling relief of aloe vera with the natural astringent properties of witch hazel. Mix 1/4 cup of pure aloe vera gel with 1 cup of alcohol-free witch hazel and 1/2 cup of warm water in a shallow basin. Soak each paw for about 1–2 minutes, then pat dry with a clean towel. This is particularly beneficial during allergy season or winter months when salt and ice can irritate paws.

Applying these remedies correctly and consistently ensures the benefits are maximized while minimizing the chance of irritation. When using ear washes, always apply with a cotton ball or pad rather than inserting anything deep into the ear canal. For a visual guide, imagine placing the cotton ball at the opening of the ear canal, gently pressing and wiping in circular motions, never pushing downward. For tooth cleaning, patience is key—start by introducing the scent and taste of the tooth powder, then build up to gentle brushing using either a soft finger brush or wrapped gauze. Keep sessions short and positive, rewarding your dog afterward.

Occasionally, even natural products can cause mild irritation, especially if your dog's skin is sensitive. If you notice redness, excessive scratching, or discomfort, discontinue use and switch to a gentler formulation. For example, if calendula causes irritation in an ear rinse, try replacing it with lavender, which is equally soothing and often better tolerated. Reluctant dogs may need a more gradual introduction with positive reinforcement—treats, praise, and short sessions can ease resistance.

It's also important to recognize when home care isn't enough. Persistent ear odor, heavy wax buildup, redness, or discharge may indicate a deeper issue requiring veterinary attention. Similarly, chronic bad breath or visible tartar could signal dental disease and necessitate a visit to a vet or professional groomer.

By integrating herbal hygiene into your routine, you create a nurturing and respectful grooming process that supports your dog's natural balance. These simple, plant-based options not only prevent discomfort but also strengthen the bond between you and your canine companion. As we move forward, we'll explore how to apply herbal care beyond hygiene, supporting your dog's wellness through calming remedies and cardiovascular support.

Combining Herbs with Prescription Medications—Safety and Timing

As more pet owners embrace a holistic approach to their animals' well-being, the intersection of herbal remedies and conventional veterinary medicine has become increasingly relevant—and complex. While herbs can offer powerful therapeutic benefits, combining them with prescription medications demands careful consideration to avoid adverse interactions. Understanding how herbs and drugs might interact, and how to time their administration correctly, is vital for ensuring your pet's safety and maximizing the effectiveness of both treatments.

Herbal supplements, like conventional drugs, can interact with the body's metabolic pathways. When used alongside prescription medications, certain herbs may either enhance or inhibit drug absorption, metabolism, or excretion. For example, St. John's Wort, often suggested for mild anxiety or depression in pets, can significantly reduce the efficacy of some prescription drugs by increasing liver enzyme activity—leading to faster drug metabolism and diminished therapeutic effect. Similarly, garlic may thin the blood, potentially compounding the effects of anticoagulant medications and increasing bleeding risk.

To help navigate the complexities, it's important to recognize common categories of veterinary medications and how they may potentially conflict with certain herbs:

Prescription Drug	Purpose	Potential Herbal Conflicts
NSAIDs (e.g., carprofen, meloxicam)	Pain and inflammation	Turmeric, willow bark (increased bleeding risk or GI upset)
Antibiotics (e.g., amoxicillin, cephalexin)	Bacterial infections	Echinacea, goldenseal (can alter gut flora or overstimulate immune system)
Anti-anxiety/behavioral meds (e.g., fluoxetine, trazodone)	Anxiety, behavioral support	Valerian, kava, chamomile (may cause excessive sedation or nervous system depression)

When using both herbs and medications, timing is a crucial safety factor. A commonly recommended practice is the "2-hour rule," which advises separating the administration of herbs and prescription drugs by at least two hours. This buffer helps reduce the likelihood of direct absorption interactions in the gastrointestinal tract and allows each substance to work without interference. For instance, if your veterinarian prescribes an anti-inflammatory at 8 a.m., give your herbal supplement no earlier than 10 a.m., ideally with food if appropriate for both substances.

Proactive communication with your veterinarian is key when exploring integrative care. It's essential to share every supplement your pet is taking, including herbal tinctures, powders, or even herbal treats. Transparency allows the vet or veterinary pharmacist to cross-check for contraindications and make personalized recommendations. Keeping track of all medications and herbs on a centralized document can facilitate these conversations. A printable "Medication and Herb Tracker" can be an invaluable tool—listing product names, dosages, administration times, reasons for use, and any observed reactions. Maintaining a log not only helps during vet consultations but offers a chronological record that can indicate patterns or emerging concerns.

To navigate discussions with your veterinarian or pharmacist confidently, consider using simple scripts such as:

- "I've started using a calming herbal tincture with chamomile and valerian. Are there any issues if my dog is also on trazodone?"

- "I'm giving my cat turmeric powder for inflammation. Is that safe to give alongside carprofen?"

- "Here's a list of everything my pet takes; can we go over it together to look for any red flags?"

Monitoring your pet closely when introducing new regimens is just as important as planning them. Watch for signs of adverse reactions, which can emerge within hours or days of starting an herb or prescription (or both). Symptoms to watch for include increased sedation or lethargy, gastrointestinal upset like vomiting or diarrhea, skin irritation, or signs of an allergic reaction such as swelling or hives.

If you see any of these changes or if your pet's behavior suddenly shifts, immediately stop administering the herb and contact your vet.

In emergency situations—such as seizures, collapse, extreme lethargy, or difficulty breathing—discontinue all supplements and medications and seek veterinary care without delay. These signs could indicate a dangerous interaction and need urgent medical evaluation.

Combining herbs with prescription medications can be safe and effective when approached thoughtfully. By understanding potential interactions, applying proper timing, and maintaining open communication with your veterinarian, you can confidently support your pet's health. The next section will further explore how to customize herbal regimens for individual pets while continuing to prioritize their overall safety and well-being.

Visual Reference Guides— Empowering Safe, Confident Decisions

When it comes to caring for your dog with herbal remedies, knowledge is important—but the ability to see what's happening can be lifesaving. Subtle changes in your dog's appearance, behavior, or body language often reveal what words can't: whether a remedy is working, needs adjusting, or should be stopped altogether. That's where visual tools come in.

In this chapter, you'll discover a series of easy-to-use, photo-driven guides and interactive decision aids designed to help you confidently navigate every stage of herbal care—from spotting early allergic reactions to knowing exactly when to call the vet. You'll learn how to compare "normal vs. abnormal" signs at a glance, use color-coded symptom charts for quick decision-making, and avoid herbs that can harm vulnerable dogs like puppies, seniors, or those with chronic illnesses. You'll also explore creative, step-by-step visual hacks for making remedies more palatable and engaging, so administering them becomes less of a battle. And when results aren't immediate, our troubleshooting flowcharts will guide you through safe, practical next steps without the guesswork.

Whether you're new to herbal care or have years of experience, these visual reference tools will empower you to act quickly, confidently, and in your dog's best interest—turning observation into prevention, and prevention into better health outcomes.

Photo Guide—Identifying Allergic Reactions and Side Effects in Dogs

Understanding how to visually recognize allergic reactions and side effects in dogs is critically important for pet owners, especially when introducing new foods, supplements, medications, or topical products. This guide offers a detailed photographic reference to help distinguish between normal and abnormal physical responses, encompassing both mild sensitivities and severe emergencies.

In our full-color visual library, you'll find real-life examples of allergic reactions ranging from subtle to extreme. Mild symptoms might include localized redness or paw licking, which are often the first indicators of irritation. Photos of dogs gently nibbling or licking their paws—sometimes mistaken as normal grooming—reveal potential signs of allergy to grass, food, or topical agents. Facial swelling is another clear warning sign. Images of dogs with puffiness around the muzzle or under the eyes showcase how even moderate reactions can escalate quickly. Hives, often seen as raised, red bumps typically on a dog's side or back, visually stand out and are another hallmark of allergic response.

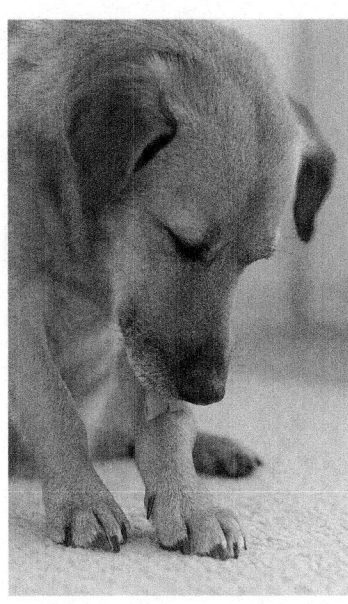

Often mistaken for grooming—watch for frequency and redness.

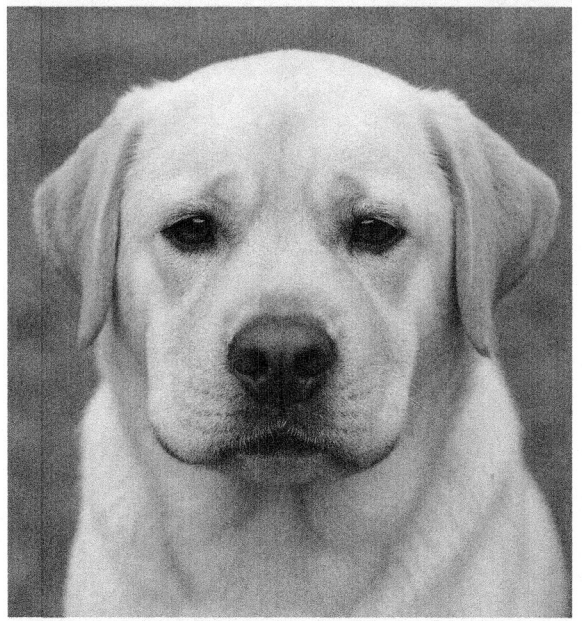

Facial swelling

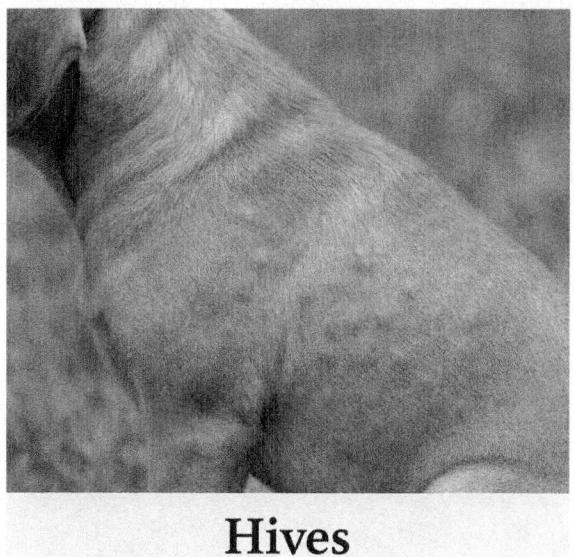

Hives

To aid in early identification, we provide "normal vs. abnormal" side-by-side comparisons for key anatomical areas commonly affected during allergic reactions. High-resolution images of a healthy dog's ears illustrate clean, pale pink interiors, whereas inflamed ears appear red, swollen, and may have dark debris. Eye condition is another revealing indicator; side-by-side images show the difference between a clear, alert gaze and irritated, watery, or runny eyes. The mouth and gums also provide clues—healthy tissue should be pink and moist, while allergic or systemic reactions can cause pale, reddened, or even discolored gums. Paws, a common hotspot for environmental allergies, are shown both in healthy condition and in states of inflammation likely caused by contact irritants or allergens.

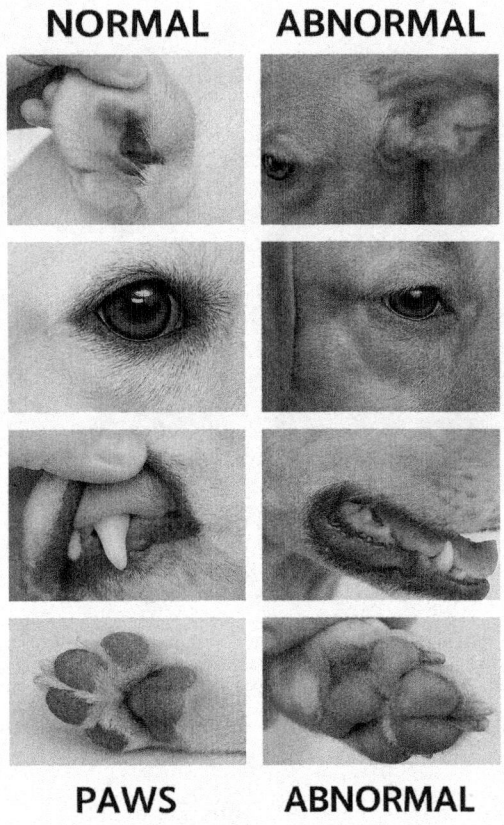

To simplify identification and action, a quick-reference symptom table links visual cues to potential causes and gives straightforward recommendations for next steps. For example:

NATURAL HERBAL REMEDIES FOR DOGS

Symptom	Possible Cause	Action
Itching after new herb	Possible ingredient allergy	Stop use, monitor for 24–48 hours
Swollen face + redness in eyes	Acute allergic reaction	Call vet immediately
Mild paw licking	Contact from grass or floor cleaner	Clean paws, monitor, consider allergy
Vomiting + Lethargy	Serious side effect or toxic ingestion	Stop product, call vet promptly
Hives + panting	Severe allergic reaction	Emergency vet care needed

This visually driven approach ensures pet parents can act fast when their dog shows signs of distress, potentially preventing more serious outcomes. By learning to spot both obvious and subtle indicators early, you'll be better equipped to keep your companion healthy and safe. In the following section, we'll delve into actionable steps pet owners can take when they suspect an allergic reaction or adverse side effect.

Visual Symptom Checker—When to Stop Herbs and Call the Vet

When giving your dog herbal remedies, it's crucial to recognize the difference between harmless side effects and serious reactions that require immediate veterinary attention. To make this easier, we've created a color-coded, visual symptom decision system that helps you quickly determine whether it's safe to continue an herbal treatment—or time to stop and call the vet.

The flowchart uses a three-color alert pathway: Green for mild, self-limiting symptoms; Yellow for signs that should be carefully monitored; and Red for warning symptoms that call for immediate veterinary intervention. Each symptom category is matched with a simple icon that represents a body system involved, like a stomach icon for digestive issues, lungs for respiratory distress, or a brain symbol for neurological changes. These visual cues allow for fast decision-making when you may be dealing with a suddenly sick or uncomfortable dog.

For example, if your dog exhibits slight, non-persistent diarrhea (represented in the chart with a yellow background and stomach icon), this is typically a Yellow-class symptom. You may choose to reduce or pause the remedy, offer supportive care (like bland food and hydration), and monitor your pet for 24–48 hours. We provide photo examples to help: a close-up image of mildly loose stool next to the Yellow-label helps you visually compare what you're seeing in real life. However, if the stool becomes watery with visible blood or your dog begins vomiting repeatedly, the photo example under the Red category (featuring bloody vomit) makes it clear this is no time to hesitate—discontinue all remedies immediately and call your veterinarian.

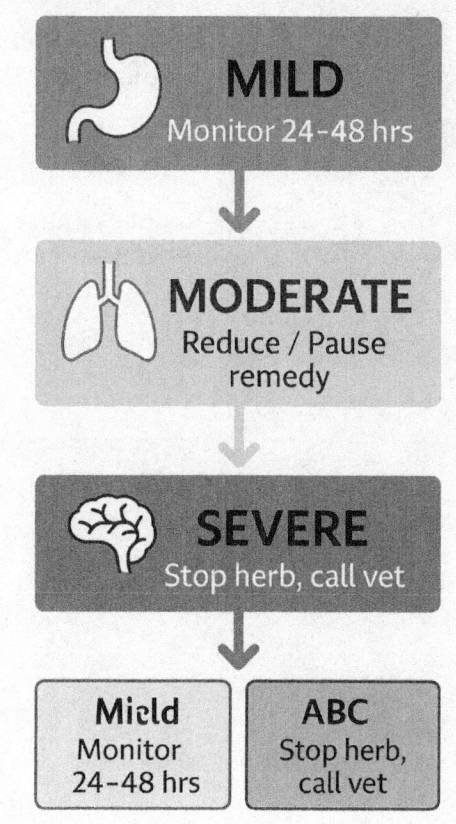

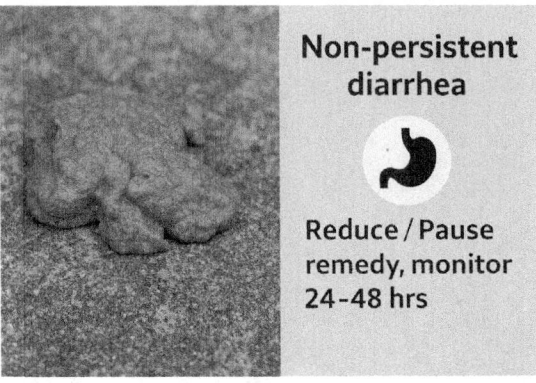

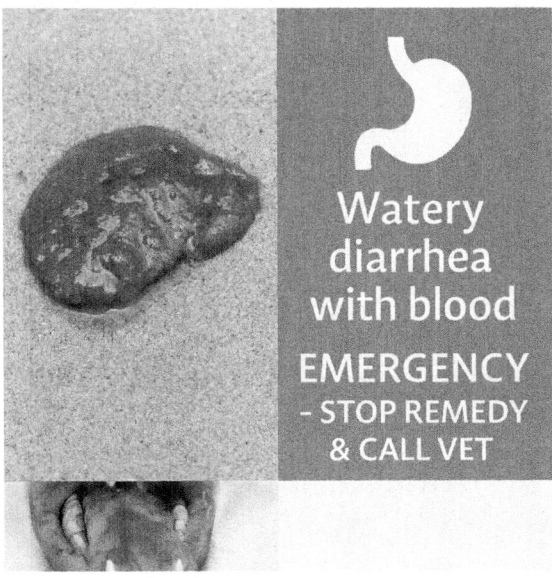

A sudden wheezing sound, shallow breathing, or excessive coughing falls under the respiratory system and is visually marked with a lung icon. Mild coughing after taking a bitter herb may be okay for observation, but labored breathing or blue gums immediately bumps that symptom into the Red zone. In the neurological category, signs such as confusion, loss of balance, trembling, or seizures are serious red flags, marked with a brain icon—and they always require emergent care.

To make this tool usable when time is critical, we offer both printable and mobile-friendly PDF versions of the chart, easily stored on your fridge, medicine cabinet, or smartphone. This downloadable checklist includes color-coded symptoms, matching photo references, and response steps—whether that means offering fluids and rest, discontinuing the herb, or calling your vet.

With herbal therapy, proactive observation is key. This visual symptom checker empowers you to respond swiftly and appropriately—ensuring that natural remedies support your dog's health, never compromise it. Up next, we'll examine the ultimate "Never Use" list—herbs that should be categorically avoided based on your dog's age, health condition, or life stage.

The Ultimate "Never Use" List—Herbs Unsafe for Puppies, Seniors, or Sick Dogs

While herbs can offer tremendous healing potential, not every herb is safe for every dog—especially when it comes to puppies, senior dogs, or those dealing with illness. These groups are more vulnerable due to underdeveloped or weakened systems, making it essential to understand which botanicals should never be used in their care. Some herbs that may benefit a healthy adult dog can prove toxic, even fatal, when given to these more delicate canines.

Garlic is one such widely debated herb. Though often promoted for its antibacterial and flea-repelling qualities, garlic contains thiosulfate, which can damage red blood cells and lead to hemolytic anemia in dogs. This risk is exponentially higher in puppies, whose organs and immune systems are still maturing. In young dogs, even small amounts may result in vomiting, lethargy, or more severe complications, making it a herb best avoided until they are fully developed—and even then, only under professional guidance.

Tea tree oil, or melaleuca, is another natural substance with a misleading reputation. Frequently touted for its antifungal and antibacterial properties in human skin care, tea tree can be extremely toxic to dogs—especially in concentrated forms. Puppies and sick or elderly dogs are particularly ill-equipped to metabolize the terpenes it contains. Ingestion, or even topical use, has been linked to symptoms ranging from muscle tremors and weakness to low body temperature and ataxia.

Pennyroyal, historically used for repelling insects and treating colds, should never be administered to dogs—particularly those with compromised health. This herb contains pulegone, a volatile compound that can severely damage the liver. Senior dogs and sick dogs often already have reduced liver function or other underlying health issues, making even small doses of pennyroyal potentially lethal.

Comfrey, despite its beneficial effects on wound healing and bone support in humans, harbors a hidden danger for dogs in the form of pyrrolizidine alkaloids (PAs). These compounds are known to cause cumulative liver damage over time. Because puppies are still developing their detoxification systems and seniors often have diminished organ function, the use of comfrey poses a long-term threat that outweighs any immediate benefits.

There are many other herbs that warrant similar caution, including those like wormwood, which can cause seizures, and yohimbe, which may severely impact heart rate and blood pressure. These and others like them should stay out of reach until more is understood about their safe dosage and application in vulnerable canine populations.

In the world of herbal remedies for dogs, what heals one may harm another. For puppies, seniors, and dogs suffering from illness, their unique physiological sensitivities require extra care in herb selection. When in doubt, always consult a holistic veterinarian before introducing any plant-based remedies. Recognizing which herbs pose dangers ensures we do no harm, while still embracing nature's healing potential for dogs of all ages.

Palatability Hacks—Make Any Remedy Dog-Approved

Getting your dog to accept herbal remedies can often feel like a game of culinary hide-and-seek. While these botanical treatments offer powerful health benefits, their distinctive tastes—whether bitter, earthy, or floral—can make them downright unappealing to the canine palate. That's where visual palatability hacks come in. By creatively disguising supplements with familiar foods, textures, and feeding methods, even the most discerning pups can be coaxed into compliance—often without realizing it.

Start with mixing herbal powders or tinctures into a flavorful base your dog already loves. A step-by-step photo guide can make this easy to replicate. For instance, one effective method shows blending powdered herbs with warm, low-sodium bone broth. The aroma and temperature of the broth help mellow the bitterness while creating a soup-like treat that most dogs find irresistible. Another approach involves inserting capsules into soft treats like cheddar cubes or sliced hot dog pieces—shown clearly in a visual series where a capsule disappears neatly inside a pliable chunk of cheese, followed by a happy dog eagerly gobbling it up.

To tailor flavor masking even further, a visual matrix of flavor pairings can be a game changer. Bitter herbs tend to blend well with umami-rich options like bone or beef broth. Floral-tasting remedies mix naturally with creamy bases such as plain Greek yogurt or goat milk. Earthy herbs often complement dense, slightly sweet foods like pumpkin purée or mashed banana. Not only does this matrix offer a visual association between herbal taste profiles and compatible edibles, but it also opens up mix-and-match opportunities depending on what you already have in your kitchen.

Beyond ingredients, consider play-based feeding tools to boost engagement. Demonstrations using silicone treat molds, interactive feeder toys, and stuffable rubber treat balls show how to transform herbal remedies into fun and edible puzzles. Pouring a yogurt-herb mix into paw-shaped treat molds and freezing them, for instance, creates lickable frozen "pupsicles." Similarly, smearing an herbal-infused peanut butter blend into a treat-dispensing ball keeps a pup engaged and licking for an extended time, improving compliance without the stress.

Even with the best efforts, not all hacks are successful on the first try. When one method fails, try adjusting the delivery: freeze the concoction, warm it slightly to enhance the aroma, or simply switch the base ingredient for something more enticing to your pet. If home remedies continually fall flat, an ""If all else fails"" sidebar notes the option of discussing your dog's needs with a veterinarian. They may recommend a compounding pharmacy that can prepare the remedy in custom flavors like chicken or peanut butter.

With a little creativity and visual guidance, transforming herbal remedies into tail-wagging treats becomes not only possible but fun. These palatability hacks empower pet parents to turn mealtime into medicine time seamlessly, paving the way to a healthier, happier pup—without the battle.

Interactive Flowcharts—What to Try Next When Results Aren't Immediate

When you're applying natural remedies, it's not uncommon to encounter moments of doubt: Is it working? Should you be seeing faster results? What if nothing seems to be changing at all? Rather than second-guessing yourself or abandoning the protocol too soon, an interactive flowchart can provide a structured, step-by-step process for evaluating and refining your approach when results aren't immediately visible.

Imagine you're a week into administering a calming herbal remedy to your dog, but you're not noticing any obvious change in behavior. This scenario is precisely where the "Remedy Troubleshooting Flowchart" comes in. At the very first decision point—"No improvement after 1 week?"—you're prompted to review three major variables: is the dosage accurate based on your pet's weight and condition? Are you using the most effective preparation method (like switching from dried herb to a more concentrated tincture)? And equally important, is your herb fresh and of high quality?

These clearly laid out decision branches help prevent unnecessary guesswork. Perhaps the tincture would be absorbed faster than capsules, or maybe increasing the frequency from twice to three times a day would help maintain consistent therapeutic levels. The flowchart includes quick-action boxes with common next steps such as, "Increase frequency?" or "Try a different herb?" Each branch is accompanied by intuitive icons and clear language to guide you confidently and safely through adjustments.

Crucially, the flowchart also incorporates sensible safety net checks. For example, if you encounter a decision point labeled "Red flag?", signs of adverse effects or worsening symptoms steer you to stop immediately and contact your veterinarian. For less concerning outcomes—such as mild effects or subtle progress—the recommendation might be to continue for an additional three days before reassessing, reducing the risk of premature changes that might obscure long-term benefits.

NATURAL HERBAL REMEDIES FOR DOGS

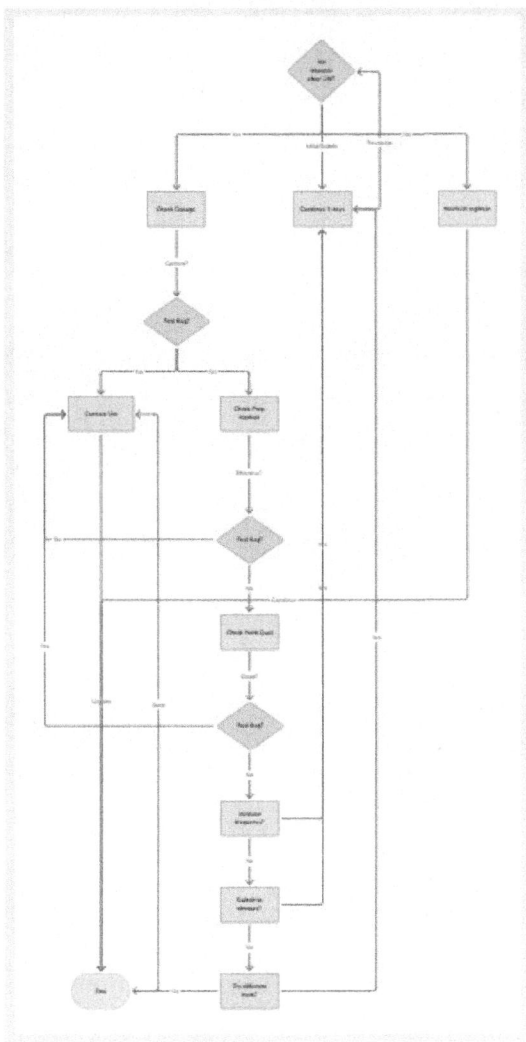

To make this tool even more accessible, we've included both printable and digital versions. A downloadable version of the "Remedy Troubleshooting Flowchart" offers a convenient reference on your fridge or clipboard. For more dynamic tracking, a QR code links to an interactive online version, complete with a treatment tracker and customizable notes. Additionally, you'll find a sample journal page designed to help you document herbal adjustments, symptom observations, and important dates. This not only supports more accurate reassessment but becomes a helpful resource when consulting with your vet.

By following a simple, visual, and data-informed process, you reduce the frustration of uncertainty and make more confident, informed decisions. Interactive flowcharts bridge the gap between theory and real-time problem-solving, ensuring that you're not just reacting—but responding deliberately—when results aren't immediate.

Real-Life Success Stories—Case Studies from Holistic Vets and Dog Parents

Nothing brings more clarity and confidence to holistic care than real-life examples of dogs who've thrived with the support of herbal protocols. Across the country, veterinarians and pet parents are witnessing firsthand how natural therapies can bring noticeable relief, improve quality of life, and build a stronger bond between humans and their canine companions. These stories are more than just heartwarming—they're rich with insights, illustrating key decision-making moments, progress milestones, and actionable takeaways.

Take Baxter, a 12-year-old Labrador Retriever who'd been struggling with age-related arthritis. His stiff joints were diminishing his once playful demeanor; daily walks became a chore rather than a joy.

His dog parent, Rachel, felt torn between increasing pharmaceutical pain meds—already causing digestive upset—and seeking a gentler solution. That's when she consulted a holistic veterinarian, who recommended a blend of turmeric and boswellia, two well-researched anti-inflammatory herbs. They began with very low doses, in line with the "start low and go slow" philosophy.

"Every dog responds differently," said Dr. Elisa Hayworth, an integrative veterinarian with over 20 years of experience. "When introducing herbs, our goal is to observe, adjust gradually, and prioritize safety above all." Just four weeks into the regimen, Baxter showed significant improvement in mobility and alertness. Alongside gentle exercise and easing into hydrotherapy sessions, the herbal protocol helped bring new life to his senior years—without compromising his digestive health.

Another case is Luna, a young mixed-breed rescue dealing with debilitating separation anxiety. Her adopter, Marco, was initially skeptical about herbal support. "Honestly, I thought herbs were just fancy salad ingredients," he joked. "But I was running out of options that didn't leave her groggy all day." Upon the advice of another holistic vet, Marco introduced lemon balm tea infusions and worked on modifying Luna's daily routine with puzzle toys and gradual departure training. The lemon balm helped take the edge off her panic, making it easier for consistent behavioral strategies to take root. By journaling daily observations and joining an online support group, Marco not only tracked Luna's progress but also connected with others on a similar journey. "Understanding the emotional side of healing—mine and hers—was huge," he reflected.

These stories aren't about overnight miracles but rather persistence, observation, and holistic thinking. Many dog parents shared similar bumps along the road: trial-and-error dosing, identifying hidden irritants (like food triggers or environmental stressors), and learning to be patient with setbacks. What ultimately helped them stay the course was a willingness to listen—to their dogs, to their chosen vets, and to their own intuition, developed over time through research and shared experience.

For instance, Rachel emphasized the value of journaling. "I wrote down everything—what Baxter ate, how much he moved, even his moods. Only then did I start to notice subtle shifts." Meanwhile, Marco's biggest lesson was learning to celebrate small wins. "The first time Luna stayed calm for ten minutes alone? We threw a mini party. It gave me the hope to keep going."

In every case, the integration of herbs into daily routines was pivotal. From creating treat-time rituals with herbal supplements to brewing calming teas as part of evening wind-downs, dog parents found creative ways to merge well-being into everyday life—even amid the chaos of work and kids. And while not every attempt went perfectly, each story uncovered powerful "what worked" versus "what we'd do differently" moments—from choosing reputable herb sources to understanding individual thresholds for dosage and delivery methods.

Collectively, these case studies underscore a simple but profound truth: healing is a journey, not a formula. With support from knowledgeable practitioners, patient observation, and a bit of trial and error, herbs can become a powerful tool in nurturing holistic health.

As we turn the page, we'll explore how to build your own holistic toolkit—balancing herbal wisdom with lifestyle strategies to meet your dog's unique needs.

Joining the Herbal Dog Community—Online Groups, Courses, and Events

Becoming part of a supportive, knowledgeable community is one of the most rewarding steps you can take on your herbal journey with your dog. Whether you're just beginning or already crafting your own tinctures and salves, connecting with others who share your passion for holistic canine care can offer education, inspiration, mentorship, and encouragement. Fortunately, the herbal dog community is thriving, with numerous online and in-person opportunities to learn and share.

Numerous active online communities bring together pet lovers, herbalists, and veterinarians who focus on botanical-based wellness for dogs. On Facebook, groups such as Herbally Healthy Pets, Holistic Dog Care: Herbal Support, and Canine Herbalism for Beginners serve thousands of members globally. These forums are often moderated by practitioners or experienced pet owners and welcome everything from newbie questions to advanced remedies. Reddit also offers a valuable resource through communities like r/herbalpets, where users regularly exchange formulas, research links, and success stories surrounding herbal care for dogs. Additionally, private forums such as The Animal Herbalism Network or the Holistic Canine Health Collective provide more curated spaces, sometimes with expert-vetted content and guest Q&As.

For those seeking structured education, several science-grounded, beginner-friendly courses are available. Look for programs led by certified veterinary herbalists, such as the Veterinary Herbal Apprenticeship Program by Dr. Randy Kidd or courses hosted by organizations like the National College of Veterinary Medicine and the Veterinary Botanical Medicine Association (VBMA). These often include modules on safe dosing, herb-drug interactions, and common condition support, making them excellent for conscientious dog owners striving for evidence-informed practices. Free and low-cost webinar series—such as those offered by animal shelters and herbal non-profits—can also be valuable, especially for those exploring complementary herbal use within veterinary care plans.

Beyond digital learning, consider attending in-person or virtual events that bring herbal dog enthusiasts together. Many cities hold seasonal herb walks and community-based meetups that welcome dog owners; these are great opportunities to learn about local plants and their uses in real-time. Annual holistic pet conferences—such as the American Holistic Veterinary Medical Association Annual Conference or Pet Wellness Summit—feature tracks explicitly focused on canine herbalism. Checking herbal apothecaries, dog-friendly co-ops, or local nature centers can uncover regional classes tailored toward both canine-specific and broader herbal learning.

Before immersing yourself in any group, course, or event, it's essential to evaluate its quality and safety. Be cautious with sources that overpromise instant cures or use language like "miracle herb" without offering evidence or encouraging individualized care. A good sign of credibility is active moderation, the presence of informed experts or practitioner input, and a respectful, science-minded tone. When considering a paid course or workshop, ask for references, syllabi, or testimonials from previous participants. Transparent goals, inclusive learning environments, and clearly listed credentials all point to worthwhile engagements.

Embracing the wider herbal dog community is more than just educational—it's empowering. When you connect with others who care deeply about their pets' wellness, you not only deepen your own understanding but also contribute to a more compassionate and knowledge-rich culture. As you build these connections, you'll find yourself more confident, inspired, and ready to support your dog's health in meaningful, natural ways.

Vet-Recommended Further Reading—Books, Journals, and Science Hubs

For dog owners, caregivers, and holistic pet enthusiasts eager to deepen their knowledge in canine herbalism, a carefully curated collection of resources can make all the difference. Whether you're just starting to explore natural remedies or are seeking science-backed information to support your progress, there are numerous veterinarian-endorsed materials that offer both insight and credibility.

A standout resource among holistic guides is The Complete Herbal Handbook for the Dog and Cat by Juliette de Bairacli Levy. Often referred to as a foundational text in natural pet care, this book has stood the test of time. Levy's practical yet compassionate approach to herbalism embraces both traditional wisdom and natural lifestyle practices, making it an essential read for anyone interested in holistic care. Although some of the information is anecdotal in nature, many veterinarians still appreciate its role in introducing concepts and natural protocols that continue to influence complementary veterinary care today.

Another highly acclaimed reference is Herbs for Pets by Gregory L. Tilford and Mary L. Wulff. Steeped in scientific inquiry and practical application, this comprehensive guide bridges tradition with modern veterinary insights. Including detailed profiles of over 150 herbs, dosage information, and safety considerations, it is often recommended by integrative veterinarians. More than just a reference, it provides context, cautionary notes, and a nuanced understanding of how herbs interact with canine physiology, making it especially useful for pet parents interested in evidence-informed herbal supplementation.

In addition to books, scientific journals offer a wealth of peer-reviewed data to support or challenge herbal practices. The American Holistic Veterinary Medical Association Journal is a go-to for professionals in the field, featuring articles on botanical medicine, case studies, and emerging trends in integrative veterinary medicine. Readers looking to build their understanding with credible, research-based insights can explore journal archives and current issues, often available to the general public through association memberships or academic libraries.

For those seeking a deeper dive into the science of herbal compounds and their effects on dogs and other animals, the National Institutes of Health's PubMed database is an invaluable hub. Simply searching terms like "canine herbal therapy" or the name of a specific herb (e.g., "turmeric in dogs") yields numerous scientific publications, many of which are open-access. PubMed's search tools allow users to filter results by type of study, publication date, and relevance, helping readers focus on high-quality, applicable research.

Complementing academic and book-based knowledge are a handful of trusted online platforms run by holistic veterinarians and experienced practitioners. Dr. Karen Becker's Healthy Pets website offers a robust catalog of articles combining conventional and integrative veterinary advice. Known for her thorough approach, Dr. Becker explores topics ranging from nutrition and herbal therapies to environmental toxins, all backed by her clinical experience and frequent citations of current studies.

Another resource gaining popularity is The Forever Dog blog and podcast, hosted by Dr. Karen Becker and animal advocate Rodney Habib. Through engaging episodes and evidence-based blog posts, the duo presents practical health strategies designed to expand canine longevity and wellness. Herbalism is woven into the broader narrative of proactive canine care, with experts frequently interviewed on subjects such as adaptogens, gut microbiota, and herbal detoxification.

Before integrating any new practice or product into your dog's regimen, knowing how to critically evaluate information is essential. A good starting point is checking author credentials—look for veterinary titles (DVM or VMD), board certifications in holistic practices, or relevant academic degrees in biology, pharmacology, or botany. Reputable authors will often cite their sources or explain methodologies, allowing readers to verify claims.

Here's a quick checklist to help discern reliable resources:

- Is the author a credentialed professional?
- Are sources cited, and are they peer-reviewed?
- Does the information reflect up-to-date findings?
- Are anecdotal stories clearly identified as such?
- Is there a balanced discussion of risks and benefits?

Learning to differentiate between anecdote and science is key in herbal medicine, where centuries of tradition often intersect with rigorous study. Balancing both can create a comprehensive understanding that honors healing wisdom while adhering to modern safety standards.

In summary, expanding your knowledge through trusted books, peer-reviewed journals, and expert media content can deepen your ability to care for your dog holistically and safely. In the next section, we'll explore how to build a home apothecary specifically tailored to your dog's needs, using the resources and insights gathered from this foundational reading.

Customizing Your Dog's Long-Term Herbal Wellness Plan

Crafting an effective, long-term herbal wellness plan for your dog doesn't require a veterinary degree—just a thoughtful understanding of your pup's individual needs, combined with a commitment to observe, adapt, and collaborate. A well-structured plan is not a rigid prescription. It's a dynamic, living roadmap that evolves as your dog ages, their environment changes, or new health goals arise. The process begins with reflection and assessment, moves into goal-setting and documentation, and continues through regular reviews and joyful collaboration with your family and trusted professionals.

Start by asking meaningful questions about your dog's current state of well-being. What is your dog's age and breed-specific susceptibility? Are they a rambunctious adolescent, a mellow adult, or an aging senior who is beginning to slow down? What is your dog's temperament—sensitive and easily stressed, or hearty and adaptable? Consider their daily environment as well. Does your dog spend time outdoors, live in an urban apartment, or share space with other animals or children? These factors will influence both herb selection and delivery methods.

Clarifying your goals is the next step in shaping a personalized plan. Preventive goals might include bolstering immunity during seasonal transitions or promoting digestive health year-round. Supportive goals address ongoing needs like mobility, stress reduction, or skin resilience. Finally, condition-specific goals target acute or chronic issues such as allergies, joint stiffness, or post-surgical recovery. Establishing a clear objective with a timeline fosters measurable progress. For example, you might define a goal like, "Reduce seasonal itching by 80% by the start of summer." Tracking this involves observing symptoms and noting flare-ups, herb usage, and even environmental factors like pollen counts.

A sample monthly check-in chart can be helpful. Rows list specific concerns (itching, energy, stool quality), while columns span four weeks to log observations and dosage adjustments. These visible progress markers can highlight what's working—and what's not—which alerts you when it's time to tweak the plan.

Wellness plans must remain fluid because your dog's life circumstances will inevitably change. Whether it's the sudden onset of arthritis, the addition of a toddler to the household, or a move from a dry climate to a humid region, your herbal approach must adapt in tandem. For instance, after relocating to a high-humidity environment, a dog prone to yeast infections may need antimicrobial or drying herbs like Oregon grape or calendula added to their baseline care. Adolescents going through hormonal shifts may temporarily require calming nervines such as skullcap, while seniors may benefit from circulatory stimulants like ginger or cognitive support from ginkgo.

Real-life scenarios serve as powerful guides. Consider a case where a midlife Labrador retriever developed fungal flare-ups after moving from Arizona to Georgia. The original wellness goal of joint support was updated to include new skin care protocols using antimicrobial rinses and internal liver support. Seasonal goals were added to prevent recurrence. Plans were reviewed more often, and dosages refined based on climate and lifestyle.

When implementing an herbal plan, include everyone who helps care for your dog. All household members—from spouses to pet-sitters—should understand herb routines, timing, and the signs of adverse reactions. One effective method is a "family herbal care calendar" posted in a shared space or synced digitally across devices. It may include daily tasks like "Add ashwagandha to dinner bowl" or weekly

NATURAL HERBAL REMEDIES FOR DOGS 147

reminders such as "Check for any hotspots." Open communication and consistent documentation not only reduce mix-ups but reinforce the partnership approach to holistic care.

Additionally, tracking tools add clarity and accountability. Printable or digital documents like the "Daily Herbal Administration Log" help reduce missed dosages. A "Symptom Tracker & Red Flag Alert Sheet" empowers caretakers to log signs like lethargy, vomiting, or changes in stool that may signal the need to temporarily stop or adjust herbal use. The "New Herb Trial Journal Page" is perfect for testing new remedies, documenting dosages, and noting any positive or negative effects during the initial six to ten days of introduction.

Organization is key for long-term success. Use the "Vet Communication Tracker" to record conversations about herbal therapies, reactions, diagnoses, or future plans. Keep emergency contact info—including holistic and conventional vets—handy via printouts near the medicine cabinet or stored digitally on a shared family drive. For modern convenience, QR codes included in this guide allow you to quickly download updated dosage calculators, digital allergy photo-reference sheets, and printable chart bundles.

To streamline herbal care into your daily routine, consider syncing your herbal log with apps like Google Calendar or Apple Reminders. Set recurring tasks for tincture administration or monthly wellness reviews. Some dog parents even print waterproof "Herbs at a Glance" reference sheets and post them near food prep stations or crates for quick guidance.

Ultimately, building and maintaining your dog's herbal wellness plan is not only about herbs—it's about mindfulness, consistency, and empowered caregiving. As your dog grows, so too will your intuition and confidence. With the right tools and an adaptable mindset, you'll be equipped to guide your beloved companion through every life stage, naturally and safely. This evolving plan will now serve as your compass, pointing the way toward vitality, comfort, and holistic support for years to come.

Printable Charts, Tracking Templates, and QR Access to Updates

Organization is the cornerstone of consistent and effective herbal care, especially when managing multiple remedies, tracking symptoms, and communicating with caregivers or veterinary professionals. To support this, a suite of thoughtfully designed printable and digital tools can make a profound difference in how smoothly herbal wellness plans are implemented day-to-day. These resources are intended to transform scattered notes and mental checklists into a streamlined, user-friendly system.

One of the most essential tools is the "Daily Herbal Administration Log," which offers a clear, structured layout for recording morning, afternoon, and evening dosages. This chart not only ensures that no dose is forgotten, but it also makes it easy to spot patterns or missed treatments—crucial when assessing effectiveness or adjusting recommendations. Another indispensable resource is the "Symptom Tracker & Red Flag Alert Sheet," which allows users to document observations over time. With designated spots to note changes in appetite, energy levels, mood, and other vital signs, this form helps identify subtle shifts that may require further attention or warrant a reevaluation of the herbal protocol.

To support the safe and measured introduction of new herbs, a "New Herb Trial Journal Page" is provided. This template enables users to document start dates, initial dosages, observed reactions, and adjustments, all in one place. Such records are invaluable for identifying allergies, sensitivities, or interactions over time. Additionally, a "Vet Communication Tracker" can be used to document consultations, questions, test results, and follow-up plans. This form is especially helpful in maintaining collaboration between holistic and conventional veterinary care providers.

To keep pace with new research, product updates, and improved tools, digital versions of all templates are available via QR codes and web links throughout the book. For instance, scanning a code on the dosage section brings up the latest dosage calculators and adjustment charts tailored to weight, species, or severity of condition. Another QR may link to an up-to-date allergy photo guide, helping users distinguish between common side effects and serious reactions. These downloadable resources make it easy to print fresh copies, access mobile-friendly formats, or share tools with family members or caregivers.

For seamless integration with everyday routines, these templates are built to work both offline and online. Readers are guided through syncing their "Herbal Administration Log" with platforms like Google Calendar or Apple Reminders—turning important dosages into scheduled, recurring alerts. Tips for printing highlight how to post a week's worth of herbal plans on the refrigerator or inside a medicine cabinet, creating visible cues that foster consistency for households managing care across multiple family members or pets.

By combining printable charts, guided tracking templates, and on-demand digital updates via QR access, this system helps users stay informed, organized, and empowered in their herbal care journey. These tools not only support better outcomes but also give peace of mind by making care plans concrete, visible, and easy to maintain. As we continue exploring practical implementation strategies, these tools will serve as reliable companions each step of the way.

Your Voice Can Help Other Dogs Thrive

Congratulations on reaching the end of this guide to natural herbal remedies for dogs! By now, I hope you feel empowered with safe, practical knowledge you can put to use in your pup's daily life.

If this book helped you—whether by saving you time at the vet, giving you new confidence to try natural remedies, or simply offering fresh ways to support your dog's well-being—I'd be honored if you could share your experience in a review.

Even a short, honest review makes a real impact:

- It helps other dog owners discover safe, reliable guidance when they need it most.

- It supports the creation of more science-backed, beginner-friendly resources like this one.

If you have a moment, your review would mean the world to me.

You can leave a review by clicking on this link or by scanning the QR code below:

Thank you for reading, for caring, and for being part of this community of thoughtful, natural-minded dog owners. Wishing you and your pup many healthy, joyful years ahead!

Conclusion

As we reach the end of this journey together, let's take a moment to reflect on the empowering transformation you've made as a committed, caring pet parent. This guide was designed with one deeply rooted purpose: to cut through the confusion and uncertainty around herbal remedies for dogs, and instead offer you a science-backed, safe, and practical path toward natural canine wellness. And with every chapter, you've moved closer to becoming your dog's most trusted herbal ally.

Over the past pages, you've learned to distinguish safe versus toxic herbs, how to build a reliable canine herbal toolkit, and source the best-quality botanicals. You've discovered preparation methods that maintain potency and safety, mastered accurate dosing with confidence, and explored how to treat everything from digestive upsets to chronic skin conditions using nature's most therapeutic plants. You've also learned how to blend holistic practices with modern veterinary care, consult user-friendly visual aids, and participate in a vibrant, supportive community that shares your dedication to your dog's wellbeing.

The biggest takeaway? You are now equipped not simply with information, but with wisdom. You can confidently choose herbs tailored to your pup's unique needs, prepare remedies that work, use safe dosages, watch for side effects, and know exactly when conventional care is still necessary. You are no longer guessing; you're acting with knowledge and purpose.

We want to acknowledge the heart behind everything you've done. You chose this path out of deep love for your dog, and that's no small thing. It takes courage to question the norm, to explore alternatives, and to step into the role of a proactive health advocate for your best friend. Celebrate the work you've put in—it matters. It's changing your dog's life.

Yet this is not an ending—it's a beginning. Herbal care is not static; it lives and evolves right alongside your dog. Keep journaling. Keep observing. Adjust the wellness plan as your dog ages or seasons shift. Continue growing—both in your knowledge and in your bond with your dog.

And you're not alone on this path. We encourage you to connect with others in this herbal wellness community. Join online groups, share your experiences, consult holistic vets, and keep discovering. There's power in community, in shared stories, and in learning from one another.

Now is the perfect time to act. Make your first herbal remedy. Review the visual guides. Print the dosage charts or tracking sheets and start using them. Don't wait—let your newfound confidence guide you into action that supports your dog's health today.

Thank you—for trusting this book, for showing up fully for your pup, and for taking the natural road with wisdom and care. Your dedication is the true remedy, and because of it, your dog will live a more vibrant, comfortable life—with the roots of wellness grounded in your hands and guided by nature. Here's to many happy, healthy years of thriving together—naturally."

Printed in Dunstable, United Kingdom